Z136.4 – 2010
Revision of
ANSI Z136.4-2005

American National Standard Recommended Practice for Laser Safety Measurements for Hazard Evaluation

Secretariat
Laser Institute of America

Approved April 22, 2010
American National Standards Institute, Inc.

American National Standard

An American National Standard implies a consensus of those substantially concerned with its scope and provisions. An American National Standard is intended as a guide to aid the manufacturer, the consumer, and the general public. The existence of an American National Standard does not in any respect preclude anyone, whether or not he or she has approved the standard, from manufacturing, marketing, purchasing, or using products, processes or procedures not conforming to the standard. American National Standards are subject to periodic review and users are cautioned to obtain the latest editions.

CAUTION NOTICE: This American National Standard may be revised or withdrawn at any time. The procedures of the American National Standards Institute require that action be taken periodically to reaffirm, revise, or withdraw this standard no later than five years from the date of publication. Purchasers of American National Standards may receive current information on all standards by calling or writing the American National Standards Institute.

Published by

Laser Institute of America
13501 Ingenuity Drive, Suite 128
Orlando, FL 32826

ISBN: #0-912035-78-1

Printed in the United States of America.

Foreword (This introduction is not a normative part of ANSI Z136.4-2010, *American National Standard Recommended Practice for Laser Safety Measurements for Hazard Evaluation.*)

In 1968, the American National Standards Institute (ANSI) approved the initiation of the Safe Use of Lasers Standards Project under the sponsorship of the Telephone Group.

Prior to 1985, Z136 standards were developed by ANSI Committee Z136 and submitted for approval and issuance as ANSI Z136 standards. Since 1985, Z136 standards are developed by the ANSI Accredited Standards Committee (ASC) Z136 for Safe Use of Lasers. A copy of the procedures for development of these standards can be obtained from the secretariat, Laser Institute of America, 13501 Ingenuity Drive, Suite 128, Orlando, FL 32826 or viewed at www.z136.org.

The present scope of ASC Z136 is to protect against hazards associated with the use of lasers and optically radiating diodes.

ASC Z136 is responsible for the development and maintenance of this standard. In addition to the consensus body, ASC Z136 is composed of standards subcommittees (SSC) and technical subcommittees (TSC) involved in Z136 standards development and an editorial working group (EWG). At the time of this printing, the following standards and technical subcommittees were active:

SSC-1	Safe Use of Lasers (parent document)
SSC-2	Safe Use of Lasers and LEDs in Telecommunications Applications
SSC-3	Safe Use of Lasers in Health Care
SSC-4	Measurements and Instrumentation
SSC-5	Safe Use of Lasers in Educational Institutions
SSC-6	Safe Use of Lasers Outdoors
SSC-7	Eyewear and Protective Barriers
SSC-8	Safe Use of Lasers in Research, Development, and Testing
SSC-9	Safe Use of Lasers in Manufacturing Environments
SSC-10	Safe Use of Lasers in Entertainment, Displays, and Exhibitions

TSC-1	Biological Effects and Medical Surveillance
TSC-2	Hazard Evaluation and Classification
TSC-4	Control Measures and Training
TSC-5	Non-Beam Hazards
TSC-7	Analysis and Applications

EWG	Editorial Working Group

The six standards currently issued are:

> ANSI Z136.1-2007, *American National Standard for Safe Use of Lasers* (replaces ANSI Z136.1-2000)
>
> ANSI Z136.3-2005, *American National Standard for Safe Use of Lasers in Health Care Facilities* (replaces ANSI Z136.3-1996)
>
> ANSI Z136.4-2010, *American National Standard Recommended Practice for Laser Safety Measurements for Hazard Evaluation* (replaces ANSI Z136.4-2005)
>
> ANSI Z136.5-2009, *American National Standard for Safe Use of Lasers in Educational Institutions* (replaces ANSI Z136.5-2000)
>
> ANSI Z136.6-2005, *American National Standard for Safe Use of Lasers Outdoors* (replaces ANSI Z136.6-2000)
>
> ANSI Z136.7-2008, *American National Standard for Testing and Labeling of Laser Protective Equipment* (first edition)

This American National Standard Recommended Practice provides guidance for optical measurements associated with laser safety requirements. The information provided in this recommended practice is intended to assist users who are entrusted with the responsibility of conducting laser hazard evaluations to ensure that appropriate control measures are implemented. Laser safety requirements and the rationale for them are specified in ANSI Z316.1 *American National Standard for Safe Use of Lasers*. The procedures and methodologies described in this recommended practice are based on requirements previously established in ANSI Z136.1. As the name implies, this recommended practice contains recommendations that will lead to the desired end result. On many occasions, there is more than one measurement approach to achieve the end result, and the recommended measurement techniques in this recommended practice should be viewed as plausible practical options, and not necessarily as the exclusive techniques to perform a given task.

This recommended practice has been published as part of the ANSI Z136 series of laser safety standards. The basic document is the ANSI Z136.1, *American National Standard for Safe Use of Lasers*. In general, this recommended practice may be used as a supplement to ANSI Z136.1 when additional details on laser safety measurements are desired.

This standard is expected to be periodically revised as new information and experience in the use of lasers is gained. Future revisions may have modified methodology, and use of the most current document is highly recommended.

While there is considerable compatibility among existing laser safety standards, some requirements differ among state, federal, and international standards and regulations. These differences may have an effect on the particulars of the applicable control measures.

Occasionally questions may arise regarding the meaning or intent of portions of this standard as it relates to specific applications. When the need for an interpretation is brought to the attention of the secretariat, the secretariat will initiate action to prepare an appropriate response. Since ANSI Z136 standards represent a consensus of concerned interests, it is important to ensure that any interpretation has also received the concurrence of a balance of interests. For this reason, the secretariat is not able to provide an instant response to interpretation requests except in those cases where the matter has previously received formal consideration. Requests for interpretations and suggestions for improvements of the standard are welcome. They should be sent to ASC Z136 Secretariat, Laser Institute of America, 13501 Ingenuity Drive, Suite 128, Orlando, FL 32826.

This standard was processed and approved for submittal to ANSI by ASC Z136. Committee approval of the standard does not necessarily imply that all members voted for its approval.

Ron Petersen, Committee Chair
Sheldon Zimmerman, Committee Vice-Chair
Robert Thomas, Committee Secretary

Notice

(This notice is not a normative part of ANSI Z136.4-2010, *American National Standard Recommended Practice for Laser Safety Measurements for Hazard Evaluation.*)

Z136 standards and recommended practices are developed through a consensus standards development process approved by the American National Standards Institute. The process brings together volunteers representing varied viewpoints and interests to achieve consensus on laser safety related issues. As secretariat to ASC Z136, the Laser Institute of America (LIA) administers the process and provides financial and clerical support to the committee.

The LIA and its directors, officers, employees, members, affiliates, and sponsors, expressly disclaim liability for any personal injury, property, or other damages of any nature whatsoever, whether special, indirect, consequential, or compensatory, directly or indirectly resulting from the publication, use of, or reliance on this document or these standards. The LIA's service as secretariat does not constitute, and LIA does not make any endorsement, warranty, or referral of any particular standards, practices, goods, or services that may be referenced in this document. The LIA also makes no guarantee or warranty as to the accuracy or completeness of any information published herein. The LIA has no power, nor does it undertake to police or enforce compliance with the contents of this document.

In issuing and making this document available, the LIA is not undertaking to render professional or other services for or on behalf of any person or entity. Nor is the LIA undertaking to perform any duty owed by any person or entity to someone else. Anyone using this document should rely on his or her own independent judgment or, as appropriate, seek the advice of a competent professional in determining the exercise of reasonable care in any given circumstances.

Participants At the time it approved this standard, ASC Z136 had the following members:

Organization Represented	*Name of Representative*
Academy of Laser Dentistry	Joel White
Altos Photonics, Inc.	Lucian Hand
American Academy of Dermatology	Mark Nestor
American College of Obstetricians & Gynecologists	Ira Horowitz
American Dental Association	Joel White
American Glaucoma Society	Michael Berlin
American Industrial Hygiene Association	R. Timothy Hitchcock
American Society for Laser Medicine & Surgery	David Sliney Jerome Garden (Alt)
American Society of Safety Engineers	Thomas V. Fleming Walter Nickens (Alt)
American Veterinary Medical Association	Kenneth Bartels
American Welding Society	Mark McLear
Association of periOperative Registered Nurses	Evangeline Dennis
Buffalo Filter	Daniel Palmerton
Camden County College	Fred Seeber
Corning, Inc.	C. Eugene Moss
Delphi Corporation	Paul Daniel Jr.
Health Physics Society	Thomas Johnson David Sliney (Alt)
High-Rez Diagnostics, Inc.	Richard Hughes
Institute of Electrical and Electronics Engineers, Inc. (SCC-39)	Ron Petersen
International Imaging Industry Association (I3A)	Joseph Greco
Kentek Corporation	William Arthur
L*A*I International	Thomas Lieb
Laser Institute of America	Gus Anibarro
Laser Safety Consulting, LLC.	Darrell Seeley
LASERVISION USA	Richard Greene
LFI International	Roberta McHatton
Lawrence Berkeley National Laboratory	Ken Barat
Lawrence Livermore National Laboratory	Robert Ehrlich
Los Alamos National Laboratory	Connon Odom
National Aeronautics and Space Administration	Guy Camomilli Randall Scott (Alt)
National Institute of Standards and Technology (NIST)	Shao Yang
North American Association for Laser Therapy (NAALT)	Raymond Lanzafame

Organization Represented	*Name of Representative*
Power Technology, Inc.	William Burgess
Rockwell Laser Industries	William Ertle
Underwriters Laboratories, Inc.	Peter Boden David Dubiel (Alt)
University of Texas, Southwestern Medical Center	John Hoopman
US Department of Health and Human Services, Center for Devices and Radiological Health	Richard Felten
US Department of Labor, Occupational Safety & Health Administration	Jeffrey Lodwick
US Department of the Air Force, Air Force Research Laboratory	Benjamin Rockwell Robert Thomas (Alt)
US Department of the Air Force, Surgeon General's Office	Scott Braley
US Department of the Army, Medical Research & Materiel Command	Bruce Stuck
US Department of the Army, US Army CHPPM	Jeffrey Pfoutz Penelope Galoff (Alt)
US Department of the Navy, Naval Air Systems Command	James Sheehy
US Department of the Navy, Naval Sea Systems Command	Sheldon Zimmerman Mary Zimmerman (Alt)
Individual Members	Robert Aldrich Prem Batra Gary Bower Richard Crowson Jerome Dennis Ben Edwards Robert Handren, Jr. Ami Kestenbaum David J. Lund Wesley Marshall Jay Parkinson Randolph Paura William P. Roach Penny J. Smalley Nikolay Stoev Paul Testagrossa Thomas Tierney Robert Weiner Anthony Zmorenski

Organization Represented	*Name of Representative*
Emeritus Members	Sidney Charschan
	David Edmunds
	James Smith
	Myron Wolbarsht

The various subcommittees that participated in developing this standard had the following members:

Measurements and Instrumentation SSC-4

Sheldon Zimmerman, Chair
Robert Thomas, Vice-Chair
Jeffrey Pfoutz, Secretary

Robert Aldrich
Prem Batra
Richard Crowson
Paul Daniel
Jerome Dennis
Edward Early
Richard Fields
Johnny Jones
Ami Kestenbaum
John Lehman
David Lund
Tom MacMullin
Wesley Marshall
Wallace Mitchell
C. Eugene Moss
John O'Hagan

Jay Parkinson
Ron Petersen
Kenneth Puckett
Benjamin Rockwell
David Sliney
James Smith
Dale Smith
Shawn Sparks
Nikolay Stoev
Paul Testagrossa
Robert Weiner
Stephen Wengraitis
Bruce Wolfe
Shao Yang
Mary Zimmerman

Laser Bioeffects, TSC-1

Bruce Stuck, Chair
David Sliney, Vice-Chair
Jeffrey Pfoutz, Secretary

Robert Aldrich
Kenneth Bartels
John Bell
Gary Bower
Clarence Cain
Francois Delori
Jerome Dennis
William Ertle
Penelope Galoff
Thomas Johnson
Charles Lin
Brian J. Lund
David J. Lund
Martin Mainster
Wesley Marshall
Russ McCally

Leon McLin
C. Eugene Moss
John O'Hagan
Ron Petersen
William P. Roach
Benjamin Rockwell
James Sheehy
Robert Thomas
Stephen Trokel
Nancy Van Cleave
Myron Wolbarsht
James Zavislan
Sheldon Zimmerman
Joseph Zuclich
Harry Zwick

Hazard Evaluation & Classification, TSC-2

Robert Thomas, Chair
William P. Roach, Vice-Chair

Robert Aldrich
Ahsan Chowdary
Jerome Dennis
Howard Donovan
Jerome Garden
R. Timothy Hitchcock
Kimberly Kantner
Martin Langlois
David J. Lund
Wesley Marshall
Leon McLin
John O'Donnell
Connon Odom
Jay Parkinson
Mary G. Payton
Ron Petersen
William P. Roach
Benjamin Rockwell
Darrell Seeley
Dale Smith
Gregory Smith
Nikolay Stoev
Bruce Stuck
Paul Testagrossa
Bill Triplett
Stephen Trokel
Karl Umstadter
Robert Weiner
James Zavislan
Sheldon Zimmerman

Control Measures & Training, TSC-4

William Ertle, Chair
R. Timothy Hitchcock, Vice-Chair
Anthony Zmorenski, Secretary

Robert Aldrich
William Arthur
Mary Baker
Ken Barat
Clarence Cain
Richard Crowson
Paul Daniel, Jr.
Jerome Dennis
Howard Donovan
Thomas Fleming
Penelope Galoff
Terence Garrison
Richard Greene
Patrick Hancock
Robert Handren
Joel Harrington
John Hoopman
Bill Janssen
Kimberly Kantner
Thomas Lieb
Susan Lohr
Tom MacMullin
Wesley Marshall
Mark McLear
C. Eugene Moss
John O'Donnell
John O'Hagan
Jay Parkinson
Mary G. Payton
Ron Petersen
Frank Rainer
William P. Roach
Benjamin Rockwell
Darrell Seeley
James Sheehy
Penny J. Smalley
James Smith
Dale Smith
David Sliney
Casey Stack
Nikolay Stoev
Bruce Stuck
Paul Testagrossa
Robert Thomas
Stephen Trokel
Robert Tucker
Robert Weiner
Jamaal Whitmore
Myron Wolbarsht
Sheldon Zimmerman

Non-Beam Hazards, TSC-5

C. Eugene Moss, Chair
Ben Edwards, Vice-Chair
Thomas Tierney, Secretary

Ken Barat
Joseph Greco
R. Timothy Hitchcock
Richard Hughes
Betty Minor
Douglas Ott

Daniel Palmerton
Ron Petersen
Penny J. Smalley
Dan Thomas
Robert Thomas
Arthur Varenelli

Analysis and Applications, TSC-7

Wesley Marshall, Chair
Robert Thomas, Vice-Chair

Robert Aldrich
Gary Bower
R. Timothy Hitchcock
Jay Parkinson
Ron Petersen
William P. Roach
Benjamin Rockwell

Dale Smith
Nikolay Stoev
Bruce Stuck
Dan Thomas
Robert Weiner
Sheldon Zimmerman
Anthony Zmorenski

Editorial Working Group, EWG

Nikolay Stoev, Chair

David Ermer
Penelope Galoff
Richard Hughes
Bill Janssen
Thomas Johnson
Ami Kestenbaum
Timothy Reed

Barbara Sams
Darrell Seeley
James Smith
Robert Thomas
Myron Wolbarsht
Mary Zimmerman
Sheldon Zimmerman

Contents

SECTION **PAGE**

SECTION PAGE

Tables

Figures

Table

Figures

Appendix F

Appendix G

American National Standard Recommended Practice for Laser Safety Measurements for Hazard Evaluation

1. General

1.1 Scope.

This document provides adequate, practical guidance for necessary measurement procedures used for classification and hazard evaluation of lasers. This document is intended to provide guidance for manufacturers, laser safety officers (LSOs), and trained laser users.

1.2 Application.

This document provides practical guidance for the measurement of those parameters necessary for the classification and evaluation of optical radiation hazards associated with lasers. Evaluation consists of comparing measured exposure levels with the appropriate maximum permissible exposure (MPE) values such as those found in the American National Standards Institute (ANSI) Z136.1 *American National Standard for Safe Use of Lasers*. The MPE is based on the ability of the laser beam or its reflection or scattering to cause biological damage to the eye or skin. Classification consists of comparing accessible radiation levels with accessible emission limits (AELs), such as those in the Federal Laser Product Performance Standard (FLPPS) 21 CFR 1040.10 and 1040.11, or the International Electrotechnical Commission (IEC) 60825-1 laser safety standard.

Generally, measurements for hazard evaluation are required only when the manufacturer's information is not available, when the laser or laser system has not been classified, or when suspected malfunctions or alterations to a system may have changed its classification or the potential hazard. For laser manufacturers and developers of lasers in the research environment, etc., measurements are especially important.

If there is a potential for exposure to laser radiation within the nominal hazard zone (NHZ) requiring the use of personal protective devices, then measurements should be attempted only by personnel trained or experienced in laser technology and radiometry. Routine survey measurements of lasers or laser systems are neither required nor advisable when the laser classifications are known, except as noted above.

This document addresses only the measurement of those parameters associated with the laser output beam. Consult ANSI Z136.1 for information pertaining to non-beam hazards associated with lasers and laser systems. Lasers or laser systems certified for a specific class by a manufacturer in accordance with the FLPPS or IEC 60825-1 standard may be considered as fulfilling all classification requirements of this recommended practice. In cases where the laser or laser system classification is not provided or where the class may change because of system alteration or the addition or deletion of engineering control measures, the LSO should ensure that reclassification of the laser or laser system is in accordance with ANSI Z136.1, the FLPPS, or IEC 60825-1.

2. Definitions

The definitions of the terms listed below are based on a pragmatic rather than an exhaustive technical approach. The terms defined are therefore limited to those actually used in this recommended practice and its appendices and are in no way intended to constitute a dictionary of terms used in the laser field as a whole. Appendix A provides a list of acronyms, abbreviations and variable symbols used in conjunction with these definitions.

accessible emission limit (AEL). The maximum accessible emission level permitted within a particular class.

accessible optical radiation. Optical radiation to which the human eye or skin may be exposed for the condition (operation, maintenance or service) specified.

alpha max. The angular subtense of an extended-source beyond which additional subtense does not contribute to the hazard and need not be considered. This value is 100 mrad for retinal thermal effects and 110 mrad for the retinal photochemical effects. Symbol: α_{max}

alpha min. The angular subtense of a source below which the source can be effectively considered as a point source. Alpha min has a value of 1.5 mrad. Symbol: α_{min}

aperture. An opening, window, or lens through which optical radiation can pass.

apparent source. The real or virtual object which forms the smallest possible retinal image.

apparent visual angle. The angular subtense (α) of the source as calculated from source size and distance from the eye. It is not the beam divergence of the source.

attenuation. The decrease in the radiant flux as it passes through an absorbing or scattering medium. Symbol: μ

average power. The total energy in an exposure or emission divided by the duration of the exposure or emission. Symbol: Φ

aversion response. Closure of the eyelid, eye movement, pupillary constriction, or movement of the head to avoid an exposure to a noxious or bright light stimulant. In this document, the aversion response to an exposure from a bright, visible laser source is assumed to limit the exposure of a specific retinal area to 0.25 s or less.

beam. A collection of light/photonic rays characterized by direction, diameter (or dimensions), and divergence (or convergence).

beam diameter. The distance between diametrically opposed points in the cross-section of a beam where the power per unit area is 1/e (0.368) times that of the peak power per unit area. Symbol: D_L

beam profile. The irradiance distribution of a beam cross-section.

beam waist. Position where the beam diameter of a focused, axis-symmetric beam is a minimum. For non-symmetric beams, there may be a beam waist along each major axis, each located at a different distance from the source.

C_A. Correction factor which increases the MPE values in the near infrared (IR-A) spectral band (0.7-1.4 μm), based upon reduced absorption properties of melanin pigment granules found in the skin and in the retinal pigment epithelium.

C_B. Correction factor which increases the MPE in the red end of the visible spectrum (0.450-0.600 μm), because of greatly reduced photochemical hazards.

C_C. Correction factor which increases the MPE for ocular exposure because of pre-retinal absorption of radiant energy in the spectral region between 1.15 and 1.40 μm.

C_E. Correction factor used for calculating the extended source MPE for the eye from the point source MPE, when the laser source subtends a visual angle exceeding α_{min}.

C_P. Correction factor which reduces the MPE for repetitive-pulsed exposure of the eye.

calorimeter. A device for measuring the total amount of energy absorbed from a source of electromagnetic radiation.

coherence. The correlation between electromagnetic fields at points which are separated in space or in time, or both. The coherence time and length are inversely related to the laser beam's spectral bandwidth. Only those lasers that are truly monochromatic are coherent, all others having a degree of coherence.

coherent. A beam of light characterized by a fixed phase relationship (spatial coherence) or single wavelength, i.e., monochromatic (temporal coherence).

collateral radiation. Any electromagnetic radiation, except laser radiation, emitted by a laser or laser system which is physically necessary for its operation.

collimated beam. Effectively, a "parallel" beam of light with very low divergence or convergence.

Condition 1. Pertains to optically aided viewing of collimated beams through telescopes or binoculars.

Condition 2. In ANSI Z136.1-2007 and this document, pertains to optically aided viewing of sources with highly divergent beams through magnifiers or eye loupes or unaided viewing with or without strong accommodation. (Condition 2 has slightly different measurement conditions in IEC 60825-1).

continuous wave (CW). In this document, a laser operating with a continuous output for a period of ≥ 0.25 s is regarded as a CW laser.

controlled area (laser). An area where the occupancy and activity of those within is subject to control and supervision for the purpose of protection from radiation hazards.

critical frequency. The pulse repetition frequency above which the laser output can be modeled as CW for the purposes of hazard evaluation. For example, for a short unintentional exposure (0.25 s to 10 s) to nanosecond (or longer) pulses, the critical frequency is 55 kHz for wavelengths between 0.40 and 1.05 μm, and 20 kHz for wavelengths between 1.05 and 1.40 μm.

D_C. The diameter, in centimeters (cm), of the collecting aperture of an optical system.

D_m. The diameter, in cm, of the measurement aperture from Table 2 (also Table 9 of ANSI Z136.1-2007) used for classification.

detector. A transducer that generates an output signal when irradiated with optical radiation.

diffraction. Deviation of part of a beam, determined by the wave nature of radiation, when it is obstructed by a surface or by a medium.

diffuse reflection. Change of the spatial distribution of a beam of radiation when it is reflected in many directions by a surface or by a medium.

divergence. In this document, the divergence is the increase in the diameter of the laser beam with distance from the exit aperture, based on the full angle between the points where the irradiance (or radiant exposure for pulsed lasers) is 1/e times the maximum value. Symbol: ϕ

NOTE: Many lasers have astigmatic divergence, i.e., have different divergences in two planes. In such cases, the divergences may be considered separately or averaged using the geometric mean. This is not consistent with the worst-case approach of IEC 60825-1.

effective energy. Energy, in joules, through the applicable measurement aperture. Symbol: Q_{eff}

effective magnification. The optical magnification used in laser safety calculations for optically aided viewing conditions. The reduction in beam diameter through an optical viewing system often increases the ocular hazard (see 4.1.4.2). Symbol: M_{eff}

effective power. Power, in watts, through the applicable measurement aperture. Symbol: Φ_{eff}

electromagnetic radiation. The flow of energy consisting of orthogonally vibrating electric and magnetic fields lying transverse to the direction of propagation. Gamma rays, X-rays, ultraviolet, visible, infrared, and radio waves occupy various portions of the electromagnetic spectrum and differ only in frequency, wavelength, and photon energy.

emission duration. The duration, in seconds, for which the laser product will emit accessible laser radiation.

energy. The capacity for doing work. Energy content is commonly used to characterize the output from pulsed lasers, and is generally expressed in joules (J). Symbol: $\boldsymbol{Q}$

exposure duration. The duration, in seconds, for which the skin or eye (as applicable) is exposed.

extended source. A source of optical radiation with an angular subtense at the cornea larger than α_{min}. See *point source*.

field of view (FOV). The full solid angle from which a detector's active area receives radiation.

flash distance. The distance at which a magnified laser diode subtends the same apparent angle as the projector lens exit port diameter (D_{exit}). Symbol: $\boldsymbol{r_f}$

focal length (*f*). The distance from the secondary nodal point of a lens to the secondary focal point. For a thin lens imaging a distant source, the focal length is the distance between the lens and the focal point.

focal point. The point toward which radiation converges or from which radiation diverges or appears to diverge.

Gaussian beam profile. A spatial profile of a laser beam which is operated in the lowest transverse electromagnetic mode, TEM_{00}. The cross section of the profile has the same shape as the normal probability curve. Many laser beams are approximated by a Gaussian profile, as a mathematical model for computing safety information.

half-power point. The time on either the leading or trailing edge of a laser pulse at which the power is one half of its maximum value, also referred to as full-width at half maximum (FWHM).

hertz (Hz). The unit which expresses the frequency of a periodic oscillation in cycles per second.

infrared. In this document, the region of the electromagnetic spectrum between the long-wavelength extreme of the visible spectrum (about 0.7 μm) and the shortest microwaves (about 1 mm).

infrared (IR) radiation. In this document, electromagnetic radiation with wavelengths which lie within the range 0.7 μm to 1 mm.

integrated radiance. The integral of the radiance over the exposure duration, expressed in joules-per-centimeter-squared-per-steradian ($J \cdot cm^{-2} \cdot sr^{-1}$).

intrabeam viewing. The viewing condition whereby the eye is exposed to all or part of a direct or specularly reflected laser beam.

irradiance. Radiant power incident per unit area upon a surface, expressed in watts per square centimeter ($W \cdot cm^{-2}$). Symbol: $\boldsymbol{E}$

joule. A unit of energy. 1 joule = 1 watt·second.

Lambertian surface. An ideal (diffuse) surface from which emitted or reflected radiance is independent of the viewing angle.

laser. A device that produces radiant energy predominantly by stimulated emission. Laser radiation may be highly coherent temporally, spatially, or both. An acronym for **L**ight **A**mplification by **S**timulated **E**mission of **R**adiation.

laser classification. An indication of the beam hazard level of a laser or laser system during normal operation or the determination thereof. The hazard level of a laser or laser system is represented by a number or a numbered capital letter. The laser classifications are Class 1, Class 1M, Class 2, Class 2M, Class 3R, Class 3B, and Class 4. In general, the potential beam hazard level increases in the same order.

laser diode. A laser employing a forward-biased semiconductor junction as the active medium.

laser safety officer (LSO). One who has the authority and responsibility to monitor and enforce the control of laser hazards and effect the knowledgeable evaluation and control of laser hazards.

light emitting diode (LED). A p-n junction semiconductor device which can be made to produce incoherent electromagnetic radiation, in the wavelength range from 0.180 μm to 1 mm, by radiative recombination in the semiconductor.

limiting angular subtense. See *alpha min.*

limiting aperture diameter. The diameter of a circle over which irradiance or radiant exposure is averaged for purposes of hazard evaluation and classification. Symbol: $\boldsymbol{D_f}$

limiting cone angle. The cone angle through which radiance or integrated radiance is averaged when photochemical effects are considered in hazard evaluation and classification. The limiting cone angle may be considered as the field of view or acceptance angle of the system for measuring radiant power or energy. Symbol: $\boldsymbol{\gamma}$

limiting exposure duration. An exposure duration which is specifically limited by the design or intended use(s). Symbol: $\boldsymbol{T_{max}}$

$\mathbf{M^2}$. Parameter that indicates how close the energy distribution in a laser beam is to that of a perfect Gaussian beam. Also called *Beam Quality*, *Beam Propagation Ratio*, or *Times Diffraction Limit Number*.

maximum permissible exposure (MPE). The level of laser radiation to which an unprotected person may be exposed without adverse biological changes in the eye or skin.

measurement aperture. The aperture used for classification of a laser to determine the effective power or energy that is compared with the AEL for each class.

minimum viewing distance. The minimum distance at which the eye can produce a focused image of a diffuse source, usually assumed to be 10 cm.

nominal hazard zone (NHZ). The space within which the level of the direct, reflected or scattered radiation may exceed the applicable MPE. Exposure levels beyond the boundary of the NHZ are below the appropriate MPE.

nominal ocular hazard distance (NOHD). The distance along the axis of the unobstructed beam from a laser, fiber end, or connector to the human eye beyond which the irradiance or radiant exposure is not expected to exceed the appropriate MPE.

numerical aperture (*NA*).

1. The sine of one half of the vertex angle of the largest cone of meridional rays that can enter or leave an optical system or element, multiplied by the refractive index of the medium in which the vertex of the cone is located. This is generally measured with respect to an object or image point and varies as that point is moved.

2. For an optical fiber in which the refractive index decreases abruptly from n_1 on axis to n_2 at the core-cladding interface, the numerical aperture is given by

$$NA = \sqrt{n_1^2 - n_2^2}$$

3. For purposes of this recommended practice, the numerical aperture is measured at the 5% of peak irradiance points (e^{-3}).

NOTE: Colloquially, NA is the sine of the radiation or acceptance half-angle of an optical fiber multiplied by the refractive index of the material in contact with the exit or entrance face. This usage is approximate and imprecise, but is often encountered.

optically aided viewing. Viewing with a telescopic (binocular) or magnifying optic. Under certain circumstances, viewing with an optical aid can increase the hazard from a laser beam. (See *telescopic viewing.*)

optical density. The logarithm to the base ten of the reciprocal of the transmittance at a particular wavelength.

$$D_\lambda = -\log_{10} \tau_\lambda ,$$

where τ_λ is the transmittance at the wavelength of interest. Symbol: $\boldsymbol{D(\lambda)}$, $\boldsymbol{D_\lambda}$ or **OD**.

optical fiber. Any filament or fiber made of dielectric materials, that guides light, whether or not it is used to transmit signals. Synonyms: *optical waveguide*; *lightguide*.

point source. For purposes of this document, a source with an angular subtense at the cornea equal to or less than alpha-min (α_{min}), i.e., $\leq$ 1.5 mrad.

point source viewing. The viewing condition whereby the angular subtense of the source, α, is equal to or less than the limiting angular subtense, α_{min}.

power. The rate at which energy is emitted, transferred, or received. Unit: watts (joules per second). Symbol: **Φ**

pulse duration. The duration of a laser pulse; usually measured as the time interval between the half-power points on the leading and trailing edges of the pulse. Symbol: ***t***

pulse-repetition frequency (PRF). The number of pulses occurring per second, expressed in hertz. Symbol: ***F***

pulsed laser. A laser which delivers its energy in the form of a single pulse or a train of pulses. In this recommended practice, the duration of a pulse is less than 0.25 s.

Q-switch. A device for producing very short (~ 1-250 ns), intense laser pulses by enhancing the storage and dumping of electronic energy in and out of the lasing medium, respectively.

Q-switched laser. A laser that emits short (~ 1-250 ns), high-power pulses by means of a Q-switch.

radian (rad). A unit of angular measure equal to the angle subtended at the center of a circle by an arc whose length is equal to the radius of the circle. 1 radian = 57.3 degrees; 2π radian = 360 degrees.

radiance. Radiant flux or power output per unit solid angle per unit area expressed in watts per square centimeter per steradian ($W \cdot cm^{-2} \cdot sr^{-1}$). Symbol: ***L***

radiant energy. Energy emitted, transferred, or received in the form of radiation. Unit: joules (J). Symbol: ***Q***

radiant exposure. Surface density of the radiant energy received, expressed in units of joules-per-square centimeter ($J \cdot cm^{-2}$). Symbol: ***H***

radiant power. Power emitted, transferred or received in the form of radiation. Unit: watts (W). Also called *radiant flux*. Symbol: **Φ**

radiometry. For purposes of this recommended practice, the measurement of infrared, visible, and ultraviolet radiation.

Rayleigh scattering. Scattering of radiation in the course of its passage through a medium containing particles whose sizes are small compared with the wavelength of the radiation.

reflectance. The ratio of total reflected radiant power to total incident power. Also called *reflectivity*.

reflection. Deviation of radiation following incidence on a surface.

refraction. The bending of a beam of light in transmission at an interface between two dissimilar media or in a medium whose refractive index is a continuous function of position (graded index medium).

refractive index (of a medium). Denoted by n, the ratio of the velocity of light in vacuum to the phase velocity in the medium. Also called *index of refraction*.

repetitive-pulse laser. A laser with multiple pulses of radiant energy occurring in a sequence.

retina. The sensory tissue that receives the incident image formed by the cornea and lens of the human eye.

retinal hazard region. Optical radiation with wavelengths between 0.4 μm and 1.4 μm, where the principal hazard is usually to the retina.

scanning laser. A laser having a time varying direction, origin, or pattern of propagation with respect to a stationary frame of reference.

solid angle. The three-dimensional angular spread at the vertex of a cone measured by the area intercepted by the cone on a unit sphere whose center is the vertex of the cone. Unit: steradians (sr). Symbol: **Ω**

source. A laser or a laser-illuminated reflecting surface.

specular reflection. A mirror-like reflection.

steradian (sr). The unit of measure for a solid angle. There are 4π steradians about any point in space.

T_1. The exposure duration (time) beyond which MPEs based upon thermal injury are replaced by MPEs based upon photochemical injury to the retina.

T_2. The exposure duration (time) beyond which extended-source MPEs based upon thermal injury are expressed as a constant irradiance.

T_{max}. The total expected or anticipated exposure duration (See ANSI Z136.1-2007 Section 3 for classification and Section 8 for intended use determination.) T_{max} may differ depending upon its use.

telescopic viewing. Viewing an object from a long distance with the aid of an optical system that increases the visual size of the image. The system (e.g., binoculars) generally collects light through a large aperture, thus magnifying hazards from large-beam, collimated lasers.

t_{min}. For a pulsed laser, the maximum duration for which the MPE is the same as the MPE for a 1 ns exposure. For thermal biological effects, this corresponds to the "thermal confinement duration" during which heat flow does not significantly change the absorbed energy content of the thermal relaxation volume of the irradiated tissue.

transmittance. The ratio of transmitted power (energy) to incident power (energy). Symbol: τ

ultraviolet radiation. In this document, electromagnetic radiation with wavelengths between 180 and 400 nm (shorter than those of visible radiation).

visible radiation (light). This term is used to describe electromagnetic radiation which can be detected by the human eye. In this document, this term is commonly used to describe wavelengths which lie in the range 400 nm to 700 nm.

NOTE: ANSI Z136.6-2005 defines visibly detectable electromagnetic radiation as having wavelengths from 380 to 780 nm.

watt (W). The unit of power or radiant flux. 1 watt = 1 joule per second.

wavelength. The distance in the line of advance of a sinusoidal wave from any one point to the next point of corresponding phase. (For example, the distance from one peak to the next.) Symbol: λ

3. Detector Properties

Measurement of laser radiation characteristics should be performed using detectors designed to accommodate the typical properties of laser beams, such as appropriate spectral and temporal responses, non-uniform irradiance pattern, and potentially high irradiance. Laser radiation detectors can generally be divided into two major categories: thermal and quantum detectors. See Appendices B and C for information on detectors.

3.1 Active Area.

The active area of the detector is the primary radiation-collecting area; optical energy striking this area will produce an electrical signal. There is a trade-off when selecting the detector size. An increase in the detector active area will allow measurements of laser beams with larger beam diameters, but will also cause increased noise and result in larger, more costly systems. One way to maximize the system throughput and signal-to-noise ratio (SNR) without increasing detector area is to carefully image the laser beam onto a small-area detector, correcting for transmission loss of the lens.

The detector's active area should be larger than the laser beam size so less than 2% is missed by the detector.

3.2 Responsivity.

Responsivity (R) is the ratio of the detector's electrical output (O) (usually in amperes or volts) to its corresponding optical power or energy input (I) (usually in watts or joules). If the detector is part of a larger system such as a power or energy meter, then the output may be read directly in units of watts or joules. The responsivity of a detector can depend on the inherent properties of the detector, the properties of the incident radiation, and the ambient conditions.

3.3 Noise Equivalent Power.

Noise equivalent power (NEP) is the optical power input required to produce a signal equal to the observed noise. In other words, NEP is a measure of the optical power that gives a signal to noise ratio of 1. NEP is calculated as follows: Given the root-mean-square (rms), noise current output (I_n), incident power (P_s), signal current output (I_s), and responsivity, $R = I_s/P_s$, NEP = I_n/R. The units are usually given as watts for power measurements (P_s, NEP) and amperes for current measurements (I_s, I_n).

Care should be exercised when interpreting NEP values. The NEP is a useful quantity for comparing similar detectors operating under identical conditions, but it should not be used as a performance measure when comparing dissimilar detectors. Factors such as chopping frequency, electrical bandwidth, and detector area influence the NEP and should be specified. A normalized NEP for unit bandwidth accounts for detector systems with different operating bandwidths and is defined as $NEP^* = NEP/B^{1/2}$ [W (Hz)$^{-1/2}$], where B is the bandwidth in hertz. Often, in the literature, NEP is actually NEP^* as defined here.

3.4 Normalized Detectivity.

Detectivity (D) is the reciprocal of the NEP. Based on sensitivity, numerically larger values of detectivity represent superior performance. A more useful parameter is the normalized detectivity [D^* (pronounced dee-star)], which normalizes the dependence of the detector area and electrical noise bandwidth. The advantage of D^* as a figure of merit is that it may be used to directly compare the performance of similar detector types with different sizes and operating bandwidths. D^* may be expressed by the following:

$$D^* = D\,((A \cdot B)^{1/2}) = ((A \cdot B)^{1/2}) \,/\, \text{NEP}\ [\text{cm Hz}^{1/2}/\text{W}]$$

where A is the detector active area in square centimeters and B is the bandwidth in hertz. Since the signal-to-noise ratio (SNR) for most detectors is also inversely proportional to $(A \cdot B)^{1/2}$, the detectivity can be interpreted as a measure of a detector's SNR normalized to an active detector area of 1 cm^2 and noise bandwidth of 1 Hz.

3.5 Spectral Responsivity.

Spectral responsivity is a measure of a detector's absolute responsivity as a function of input wavelength. This is commonly depicted on a graph called a spectral responsivity curve as shown in Figure 1. This curve can be used to evaluate a detector's suitability for use with a particular source for a given application. Many detectors are categorized according to their wavelength response characteristics, for example, UV, visible, and IR detectors.

In general, spectral responsivity is determined by the inherent optical absorptance characteristics of the detector material, along with any surface coatings or window materials. Many quantum detectors such as silicon (Si), germanium (Ge), indium gallium arsenide (InGaAs), and gallium arsenide (GaAs) exhibit strong wavelength dependence. Thermal detectors, on the other hand, have a relatively *flat* spectral responsivity, which implies that they respond uniformly over a wide wavelength range. When performing measurements, the spectral distribution of the laser source should be known and be within the spectral responsivity range of the detector. It is also important to note that the detector spectral responsivity will vary with detector temperature, spatial uniformity, and other properties such as the window material and thickness that are not inherent to the detector material.

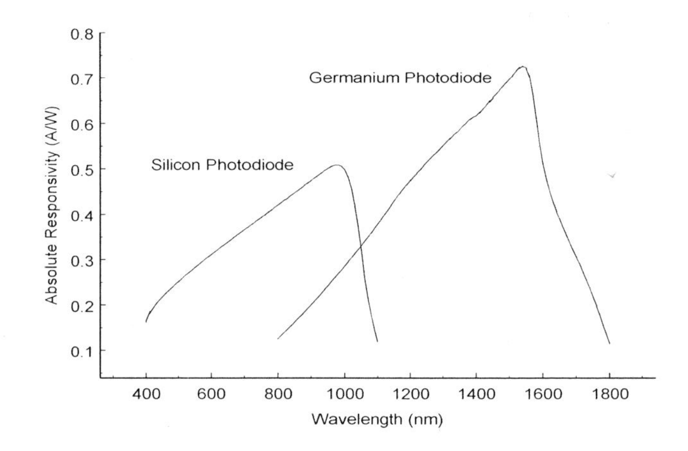

Figure 1. Spectral Responsivities of Silicon and Germanium Photodiodes

3.6 Spatial Uniformity.

The variation of responsivity as a function of position on the detector surface is called spatial uniformity. Spatial uniformity is usually measured by scanning a small, constant-power laser beam across the detector's surface while monitoring its response. Typical results for two similar detectors are shown in Figure 2. For laser beams that have non-uniform irradiance profiles or are smaller than the detector surface, detectors that have poor spatial uniformity will contribute to measurement error. Appendix C lists the worst-case spatial uniformity range for several detector types.

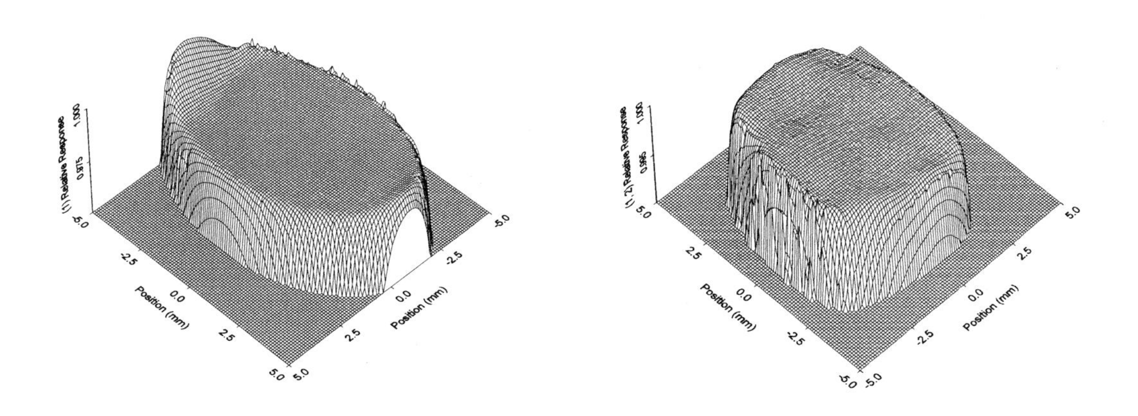

Figure 2. Detector Spatial Uniformity

3.7 Response Linearity.

If the detector output has a linear relationship with respect to the incident laser power or energy, that is, the responsivity is constant, then the detector is said to be linear. If the responsivity increases with the increase of the input, the detector has a positive nonlinearity (or supralinearity); and if the responsivity decreases with the increase of the input, the detector has a negative nonlinearity (or saturation). Positive nonlinearity is typically seen in photodiodes with indirect recombinations. Negative nonlinearity is typically caused by direct recombination in photodiodes, or when the input reaches a point where the detector or its associated electronics are saturated (especially applicable to quantum detectors). Negative nonlinearity is also seen where nonlinear thermal processes, such as convective or radiative heat transfer in thermal detectors, begin to dominate. Nonlinearity can also be caused by electrical effects such as range discontinuity (for example, amplifier and resistance offsets when using different ranges on a meter) and impedance mismatches. Nonlinearity of a detector is a potential source of uncertainty. However, nonlinear detectors can still be used for accurate measurements if the nonlinearity is quantified.

3.8 Power/Energy Range.

When using a laser power/energy meter, the proper scale or range should be selected. It is usually good practice to start on the highest range for which the measurement is expected, and then to work to lower ranges. Some instruments should have the "zero" reading adjusted on each range prior to the final measurement.

3.9 Damage Threshold.

The minimum irradiance or radiant exposure required to cause damage to a detector is called the damage threshold for that detector. It is best to avoid damage to the detector since it causes a permanent change in detector responsivity, and also may result in the need for repair or replacement of the detector. The manufacturer usually specifies damage threshold values in terms of $W \cdot cm^{-2}$ for CW applications or $J \cdot cm^{-2}$ for pulsed applications. The damage thresholds are approximate and may vary from unit to unit even for the same model of detector. Damage thresholds may be dependent on wavelength, pulse duration, repetition rate, and spot size. To ensure that the laser beam to be measured does not exceed the damage threshold it is desirable to calculate the anticipated irradiance or radiant exposure. These calculations require knowledge of the parameters of the laser beam: cross-sectional shape (circular, rectangular, etc.), diameter (or dimensions if beam is not circularly symmetric), total power or energy, and irradiance profile (if available).

If the beam profile has circular symmetry and is predominantly Gaussian, then the peak irradiance or radiant exposure of the beam can be calculated in a straightforward manner. Divide the total power or energy of the beam by the cross sectional area at the 1/e points (the points where the irradiance has dropped to a value 1/e [approximately 0.368] times the maximum). If the beam has irregular regions of high irradiance or radiant exposure, known as "hot spots," or an asymmetrical irradiance profile, then the calculations are more difficult and should be handled individually. If in doubt, test samples coated with the same absorbing material as the detector should be exposed to the laser beam before using the actual detector.

3.10 Detector Response Time.

The response time or "speed" of a detector is typically characterized by its stated time constant, which is normally supplied by the manufacturer. The time constant for thermal detectors and some quantum detectors is usually determined by measuring the time required for the detector output to decrease to a factor of 1/e from a starting value once laser radiation exposure has been discontinued. This measurement is based on the assumption that the decay of the detector output is exponential and has a single exponential coefficient. Quantum detectors generally have much shorter time constants than thermal detectors and, consequently, are the predominant type of detector for temporal characterization of laser radiation pulses. The speed of quantum detectors is often measured by performing impulse response measurements to determine their rise times and impulse response durations.

A detector's response time is usually a function of more than just the detecting element; so, when determining response time, the "detector" may include amplifiers, oscilloscopes, and other associated electronics.

3.11 Pulse Repetition Effects.

Many radiometers that measure individual pulses have a recycle time that is determined either by the detector or the indicator electronics. Therefore, repetitive pulses cannot be measured if the pulse repetition frequency (PRF) exceeds the capability of the detector or meter. Pyroelectric detectors that use optical choppers cannot be used to measure pulsed lasers because part of the radiation will strike the chopper wheel and will not expose the detector to the correct frequency. If a fast detector is not available, a measurement of the pulse repetition frequency and the total energy or average power of a pulse train can be used to compute the average pulse energy. Detector saturation levels must be considered when average power measurements are used for pulsed sources.

3.12 Background or Stray Radiation.

Measurements are often made when unwanted optical radiation is in the field of view of the test detector. Sunlight, room light, flashlamp light, or other stray radiation from the surroundings may result in offsets, which will affect the accuracy of the results. Many commercially available detector systems may be nulled or zeroed before performing measurements to compensate for offsets. Narrow bandpass optical filters transmitting at the laser's wavelength can be used to minimize background or stray radiation. The relative magnitude of the background radiation compared with the laser output determines the amount of effect on the measurement.

3.13 Environmental Sensitivity.

Some detectors may be susceptible to noise, vibration, electromagnetic interference, humidity or temperature variations that will affect the measurement results. These effects should be kept in mind when performing measurements.

3.14 Field of View and Alignment.

Field of view (FOV) is the full solid angle from which the detector's active area receives radiation. Many detection systems use a window or lens situated between the detector and the energy source. The FOV is determined by the detector's active area, the area of the window, lens, or aperture, and the distance from detector surface to the window, lens, or aperture. Alignment may be more difficult for detectors that have a narrow field of view.

3.15 Radiometric Instrument Detector Systems.

In practice, laser power/energy meters and irradiance or radiant exposure meters are designed and calibrated with the limitations of the component detector as described in paragraphs 3.1 through 3.14. The detector is enclosed in a detector unit and connected to an electronic readout system. Combined limitations of the detector and the readout electronics will limit the manufacturer's specifications for the complete instrument. It is critical that the user carefully read the specifications of the actual instrument prior to use. The angular response is generally designed to be Lambertian (cosine response), and if not specified, most detectors have a limiting cone angle of acceptance that the user can determine by sample measurements. An added, limiting aperture or a hood with a limited cone angle of acceptance can be fabricated by the user for use in laser safety measurements, but the modified system should be fully characterized before use.

3.16 Calibration and Measurement Uncertainty.

Calibration and measurement uncertainties are associated with all radiometric measurements. Factors such as non-ideal properties of the sensor, the nature of the source, background radiation, environmental conditions, and calibration procedures contribute to measurement uncertainty. The terms *precision* (also referred to as *variability*) and *bias* are preferred for describing measurement uncertainty. *Precision* quantifies the magnitude of a random effect whereas *bias* quantifies the magnitude of a systematic effect. The magnitude of a random effect can be reduced by averaging a group of measurements while a systematic effect can not. Normally, by a process of calibration referenced to a detector standard, systematic uncertainty can be corrected or used as part of calibration offset. (B.N. Taylor, C.E. Kuyatt (1994), *Guidelines for Evaluating and Expressing the Uncertainty of NIST Measurement Results*, NIST Technical Note 1297.)

4. Laser Classification and Hazard Evaluation

4.1 Background.

The following basics of hazard evaluation should be reviewed prior to making measurements to ensure that the resulting measured data will be useful for assessing hazards.

4.1.1 Exposure Duration. There are several exposure durations to consider when conducting classification or hazard analysis. The limiting exposure duration is represented by the symbol, T_{max}. These exposure durations will determine exposure limits along with measurement and limiting aperture diameters. Tables 1 and 2 list the recommended limiting exposure durations for these conditions. Longer or shorter exposure durations may be used depending on the design or intended use of the system. Devices must satisfy the MPE or AEL requirements (as applicable) for all time durations up to T_{max}.

4.1.2 Limiting Aperture Diameter (D_f). The limiting aperture diameter (D_f) is the maximum diameter of a circle over which power or energy can be averaged. For visible or near infrared lasers that can primarily cause damage to the retina, this is simply the maximum size of the pupil, defined as 0.7 cm. For lasers that are not in this wavelength region, the concept of the limiting aperture still holds the same meaning. The limiting aperture is a function of both the laser wavelength and the exposure duration. Table 1 shows a list of limiting aperture diameters and is derived from ANSI Z136.1-2007.

In any measurement procedure used in a hazard analysis, it is important to keep in mind that the end goal is to determine the amount of power or energy that will be transmitted by this aperture. The power or energy transmitted by this aperture is the value to be compared directly to an accessible emission limit (AEL). For example, since the eye can focus all laser energy in the retinal hazard wavelength region entering the pupil to a small spot on the retina, the actual size of the beam, if smaller than the pupil, is irrelevant. This is a very important concept in evaluating the hazards and for hazard classification of a laser.

4.1.3 Effective Power or Energy (Φ_{eff} or Q_{eff}). For any laser hazard evaluation, the appropriate measurement aperture is selected and the power is measured through that aperture. This effective power or energy is the value used to compare to the AEL to determine the laser classification and associated hazards. However the *total* power or energy (Φ_0 or Q_0) is incorporated into the formula for NOHD computations.

4.1.4 Effect of Optically Aided Viewing. ANSI Z136.1-2007 states that both unaided and optically aided viewing conditions shall be considered for lasers between 302 nm and 2.8 μm. Viewing aids do not transmit a significant portion of the total beam power or energy at wavelengths outside this spectral region; therefore the laser beam would not be as hazardous with viewing optics as without their use. For hazard evaluation, the hazards from viewing optics should be considered for outdoor operations. Other devices normally encountered indoors, such as fiber optic connectors, may involve the use of optical aids, e.g., eye loupes. When the specific type of optics is unknown, standard 7×50 binoculars provide a convenient means for evaluating the hazards with telescopic optics. To account for additional hazards due to eye loupes or hand magnifiers, the measurement aperture is placed closer to the source. When specific optical devices are expected to be encountered, these specialized optics should be considered.

4.1.4.1 Measurement Apertures. The measurement apertures listed in Table 2 are to be used when determining the effective power or energy for classification. The measurement aperture for unaided viewing is equal to the limiting aperture. For optically aided viewing, two viewing conditions are considered. For Condition 1 in the classification criteria (see Table 2), standard 7×50 binoculars (magnification of 7 and 50-mm objective lens diameter) are used when determining the aided viewing condition for classification. The measurement aperture for aided viewing with standard 7×50 binoculars is approximately equal to the limiting aperture multiplied by 7 (50 mm for the retinal hazard region, otherwise, see Table 2). For hazard evaluation involving other optical systems, the measurement aperture for aided viewing is the limiting aperture multiplied by the effective magnification (see 4.1.4.2). Condition 2 in the classification criteria considers unaided viewing. A measurement aperture of 7 mm in diameter is placed at a distance of 10 cm from the source to account for this hazard. (See Table 2 and ANSI Z136.1-2007 for this distance).

NOTE: Values in Tables 1 and 2 match Tables 8 and 9 of ANSI Z136.1-2007. If a newer version of the ANSI Z136.1 is available, then limiting and measurement apertures should be taken from the newer document.

4.1.4.2 Effective Magnification. The effective magnification is related to the increase in hazard from an optical viewing device. The beam diameter of a laser can be reduced by the magnification of an optical system. When the exit beam diameter from the optical system is larger than the limiting aperture, the effective magnification is the normal magnification. However, when the exit beam diameter is smaller (either from a small original beam diameter or from a higher magnification system), the effective magnification is reduced from the normal magnification by the ratio of the exit beam diameter to the limiting aperture diameter.

NOTE: When the original beam diameter is equal to or smaller than the limiting aperture, the effective magnification is 1. When the original beam diameter is larger than the entrance aperture of the optics, the exit beam diameter is equal to the entrance aperture divided by the normal magnification. Otherwise, the exit beam diameter is equal to the beam diameter divided by the normal magnification.

4.1.5 Maximum Permissible Exposure (MPE). The MPE (see Section 2) is based on a simplified model of actual biological data collected from many studies. If the laser is capable of producing a higher irradiance or radiant exposure than the MPE, the laser can pose a hazard. The higher the output is over the MPE, the greater the hazard presented.

Table 1
Limiting Apertures (Irradiance and Radiant Exposure) and Limiting Cone Angles γ (Radiance and Integrated Radiance) for AEL Determination and Hazard Evaluation

Spectral Region (μm)	Duration† (s)	Aperture Diameter (mm) Eye	Skin
0.180 to 0.400	10^{-9} to 0.3	1.0	3.5
	0.3 to 10*	$1.5\,t^{0.375}$	3.5
	10 to 3×10^4	3.5	3.5
0.400 to 1.400	10^{-13} to 3×10^4	7.0	3.5
1.400 to 10^2	10^{-9} to 0.3	1.0	3.5
	0.3 to 10*	$1.5\,t^{0.375}$	3.5
	10 to 3×10^4	3.5	3.5
10^2 to 10^3	10^{-9} to 3×10^4	11.0	11.0
		Limiting Cone Angle, γ (mrad)	
0.400 to 0.600	0.7 to 100	11	
	100 to 10^4	$1.1\,t^{0.5}$	
	10^4 to 3×10^4	110	

* Under normal conditions these exposure durations would not be used for hazard evaluation.

† For guidance on exposure durations less than 10^{-13} seconds, see ANSI Z136.1-2007. Since different limiting and measurement apertures apply for pulsed versus CW exposures, the aperture for Rule 1 is determined from the duration of a single pulse. For Rule 2, the potential exposure for all exposure durations, T, less than or equal to T_{max} is compared with the MPE for T with the corresponding limiting aperture determined from T. For Rule 3, the aperture is determined from the duration of a single pulse, but not less than t_{min}. The energy from pulses contained within exposure duration t_{min} is considered a single pulse for Rule 3. Information on these Rules is available in Section 8.2.3 of ANSI Z136.1-2007.

NOTE: The wavelength region λ_1 to λ_2 means $\lambda_1 \le \lambda < \lambda_2$ μm, e.g., 0.315 to 0.400 μm means $0.315 \le \lambda < 0.400$ μm. Additionally, the exposure duration region t_1 to t_2 means $t_1 \le t < t_2$ s, e.g., 0.3 to 10 s means $0.3 \le t < 10$ s.

Table 2
Measurement Apertures for Laser Classification*

			Condition 1		Condition 2	
Spectral Region** (μm)	Exposure Duration† (s)	Optics Transmission	Aperture Diameter§ (mm)	Measurement Distance (cm)	Aperture Diameter (mm)	Measurement Distance# (cm)
0.180 to 0.302	10^{-9} to 0.3 0.3 to 10 10 to 3×10^4	0%††	N/A	N/A	1.0 $1.5\ t^{0.375}$ 3.5	10
0.302 to 0.4	10^{-9} to 0.3 0.3 to 10 10 to 3×10^4	70%	7.0 $11\ t^{0.375}$ 25.0	200	1.0 $1.5\ t^{0.375}$ 3.5	10
0.4 to 1.4	10^{-13} to 3×10^4	90%	50.0	200	7.0	10
1.4 to 2.8	10^{-9} to 0.3 0.3 to 10 10 to 3×10^4	70%	7.0 $11\ t^{0.375}$ 25.0	200	1.0 $1.5\ t^{0.375}$ 3.5	10
2.8 to 10^2	10^{-9} to 0.3 0.3 to 10 10 to 3×10^4	70% (<4.0 μm) 0%†† (≥4.0 μm)	N/A	N/A	1.0 $1.5\ t^{0.375}$ 3.5	10
10^2 to 10^3	10^{-9} to 3×10^4	0%††	N/A	N/A	11.0	10

* These apertures are used for the measurement of optical power or energy for the purpose of laser classification (see Section 3.3 of ANSI Z136.1-2007). The standardized measurement apertures and distances actually simulate many viewing conditions and do not necessarily refer only to viewing at those measurement distances.

** Condition 1 does not apply for lasers having wavelengths exceeding 2.8 μm since most telescopic optics do not transmit beyond 2.8 μm; however, the IEC 60825-1 applies Condition 1 to lasers that have wavelengths up to 4.0 μm in consideration of special purpose telescopes that have transmission over an extended spectral range.

† For guidance on exposure durations less than 10^{-13} seconds see Section 8.2.2 of ANSI Z136.1-2007. Exposure durations between 0.3 s and 10 s would not normally be used for classification.

§ Under use conditions, when laser output is intended to be viewed with optics (excluding ordinary eyeglasses) or the Laser Safety Officer determines that there is a reasonable probability of accidental viewing with optics, the apertures listed in Table 1 for hazard evaluation apply to the exit beam from the particular optical instrument being considered. For situations where the default conditions do not apply, refer to the hazard analysis techniques in the examples in B6.4.3 in Appendix B of ANSI Z136.1-2007.

The default measurement distance for Condition 2 in the IEC 60825-1 is 7 cm.

†† Transmission at these wavelengths is low enough that Condition 2 is more restrictive.

NOTE: The wavelength region λ_1 to λ_2 means $\lambda_1 \leq \lambda < \lambda_2$ μm e.g., 0.315 to 0.400 μm means $0.315 \leq \lambda < 0.400$ μm.

4.1.6 Accessible Emission Limit (AEL). The Class 1 AEL is calculated by multiplying the ocular MPE by the area of the limiting aperture for the eye. The AELs for other classes are either based on the Class 1 AEL for specific viewing conditions, or on other biological hazards. The worst case of unaided and optically aided viewing conditions determines the class of the laser. Only the effective power or energy (that power or energy that is transmitted by the measurement aperture) is compared with the AEL for each class. When the measurement aperture is larger than the limiting aperture, due to the potential use of optical aids, the transmittance of these optics is included (see Table 2) for hazard evaluation and classification.

4.1.7 Apparent Source. The apparent source is the real or virtual object which forms the smallest possible retinal image. For the classification and hazard analysis of an extended source laser, it is critical to know the dimensions and location of the apparent source, or the angular subtense of the source. For small-source lasers, the apparent source is usually assumed to be located far behind the output aperture of the laser, unless there is an external beam waist. The effective magnification of an optical device can influence the location and/or size of the apparent source. If the location and size of the apparent source cannot be determined, using a point source in the evaluation will provide a conservative result.

4.1.8 Apparent Visual Angle (α). The apparent visual angle (angular subtense) of the source is calculated as the physical size of the apparent source divided by its distance from the eye or viewing optics. For classification, the apparent source size is determined from a specific distance provided in Table 2 (10 cm for unaided viewing). Since the normal human eye images only in the retinal hazard region (400 nm-1.4 μm), angular subtense is defined only over this spectral band. The size of the retinal image produced when viewing a source of optical radiation is especially important in assessing the biologic effect from viewing a direct laser beam or a diffuse laser reflection. The dimensions of the retinal image are related to the apparent visual angle of the source. The apparent visual angle is important only if it exceeds α_{min}. For extended sources, non-uniform irradiance can affect the ocular hazards from the source and the classification. Measurement of apparent visual angle is covered in Section 5.5.

4.1.9 Measurement Distance. The measurement distance is the distance from the output aperture or apparent source of the laser at which the effective power or energy is measured through apertures placed at specified distances in accordance with Table 2 for classification except for the case of a beam with an external waist located at a farther distance. In those cases, the specified aperture is placed at the beam focus. For a hazard evaluation, the measurement distance is determined by the circumstances analyzed. For the purposes of classification there are two measurement distances to consider, one for unaided viewing and one for telescopic viewing. For information on how to determine measurement distance, see Table 2 and Appendix D, Section D 11.2.

NOTE: The measurement apertures and distances provided in Table 2 were current at the time of publication; however, in some specialized cases, the measurement distances for Condition 2 could be revised in the future, and the reader is advised to check with the most current ANSI Z136.1 or IEC 60825-1 standard.

4.1.10 Limiting Cone Angle (γ). For photochemical effects, the radiance or integrated radiance is averaged over γ for comparison with the MPE. If the angular subtense α of the source is larger than γ, then only the radiant energy within γ is applicable for comparison with the MPE. If the angular subtense α of the source is smaller than γ, the radiance or integrated radiance of the source is averaged over γ before comparison with the MPE.

NOTE: For measurements of single point sources, where $\alpha < \gamma$, irradiance or radiant exposure measurements will provide sufficient information to compute average radiance or integrated radiance values for comparison with the MPE. Therefore, it is only necessary that the field of view be larger than α to evaluate photochemical hazards, and need not be well-defined.

4.1.11 Radiance Measurements. Radiance ("radiometric brightness") is a primary radiometric quantity used in the assessment of retinal hazards from lamps and lighting systems (see ANSI RP27.1, RP27.2, and RP27.3), but is not routinely used in laser safety except for assessing viewing of laser radiation sources of very large angular subtense α. All thermal MPEs and AELs for angular subtenses greater than α_{max} are a constant radiance and all photochemical MPEs and AELs can be expressed as a constant radiance. Radiance is a radiometric quantity of particular importance for assessing retinal hazards since retinal irradiance is directly proportional to source radiance for all viewing distances where the source appears as an extended source. Radiance is frequently referred to as the "radiometric invariant," since it can be measured at the source or at any distance and remains constant. For example, for a large, uniform diffuse reflection, the source size remains constant, while the irradiance decreases inversely as the square of the distance. Since the solid angle Ω subtended by the source decreases inversely as the square of the distance, the radiance remains constant at different viewing distances. [The solid angle decreases inversely as the square of the distance because the apparent visual angle (linear angle) decreases inversely as the distance.]

To calculate radiance from measured values, the received irradiance is averaged over both a limiting aperture, and also a field-of-view. In conventional radiometry, one always chooses an angular field of acceptance that is smaller than the source. However, for some laser safety measurements, such as for photochemical MPEs, the angular field of acceptance, [i.e., the limiting cone angle (γ)] is specified for a given exposure duration.

4.2 Laser Classification Schemes.

4.2.1 Hazard Classes. Laser hazard classifications are used to quantify the level of hazard inherent in a laser system and the extent of safety controls required. These range from Class 1 lasers (which are safe for direct beam viewing under most conditions) to Class 4 lasers (which are the most hazardous and require the most rigid controls). Hazard classification is based upon the worst case of unaided or 5 cm aided viewing conditions. For a comparison of ANSI Z136.1 and IEC 60825-1 classifications, refer to Appendix H of ANSI Z136.1-2007. A description of the ANSI and the IEC laser classification schemes follows (the FLPPS has its own classification scheme as well as allowing use of IEC classifications.)

4.2.1.1 ANSI Laser Classes. ANSI Z136.1-2007 includes the following classes of lasers and laser systems.

4.2.1.1.1 Class 1 and Class 1M Lasers and Lasers Systems. Class 1 and Class 1M are delineated as follows.

4.2.1.1.1.1 Any laser, or laser system containing a laser, that cannot emit accessible laser radiation levels during operation in excess of the applicable Class 1 AEL for any emission duration within the maximum duration inherent in the design or intended use of the laser or laser system is a Class 1 laser or laser system during operation. The maximum exposure duration is assumed to be no more than 30,000 s, except for infrared systems not intended to be viewed ($\lambda > 700$ nm) where 100 s is used. The hazard class strictly applies to emitted laser radiation hazards and not to other potential hazards (see Section 7 in ANSI Z136.1-2007, Non-Beam Hazards).

4.2.1.1.1.2 Lasers or laser systems intended for a specific use may be designated Class 1 by the LSO on the basis of that specific use with a limiting exposure duration of T_{max} less than 100 s, provided that the accessible laser radiation does not exceed the corresponding Class 1 AEL for any emission duration within the maximum duration inherent in that specific use.

4.2.1.1.1.3 Any laser or laser system that cannot emit during operation accessible laser radiation levels in excess of the applicable Class 1 AEL under the conditions of measurement for the unaided eye, but exceeds the Class 1 AEL for telescopic viewing (Table 9 in ANSI Z136.1-2007) is a Class 1M laser or laser system provided that it does not exceed the Class 3B AEL for any emission duration within the maximum duration inherent in the design or intended use of the laser or laser system. The maximum exposure duration is assumed to be no more than 30,000 s.

4.2.1.1.2 Class 2 and Class 2M Visible Lasers and Laser Systems. Class 2 and 2M lasers and laser systems are visible (400 to 700 nm) CW and repetitive-pulse lasers and laser systems which can emit accessible radiant energy exceeding the appropriate Class 1 AEL for the maximum duration inherent in the design or intended use of the laser or laser system, but not exceeding the Class 1 AEL for any applicable pulse (emission) duration < 0.25 s and not exceeding an accessible average radiant power of 1 mW. Class 2M lasers and laser systems pose the same ocular hazards to the unaided eye as Class 2, but are potentially hazardous when viewed with optical aids.

4.2.1.1.2.1 Any laser or laser system that cannot emit during operation accessible laser radiation levels in excess of the applicable Class 2 AEL under the conditions of measurement for the unaided eye, but exceeds the Class 2 AEL for optically-aided viewing (Table 9 in ANSI Z136.1-2007) is a Class 2M laser or laser system, provided that it does not exceed the Class 3B AEL for any emission duration within the maximum duration inherent in the design or intended use of the laser or laser system. The maximum exposure duration is assumed to be no more than 0.25 s.

4.2.1.1.3 Class 3 (3R and 3B) Lasers and Laser Systems. Class 3 lasers have two categories, 3R and 3B.

4.2.1.1.3.1 Class 3R lasers and laser systems include lasers and laser systems which have an accessible output between 1 and 5 times the Class 1 AEL for wavelengths shorter than 400 nm or longer than 700 nm, or greater than the Class 1 AEL but less than 5 times the Class 2 AEL for wavelengths between 400 and 700 nm.

NOTE: Products can be classified as Class 1M and Class 2M even if their output exceeds Class 3R.

4.2.1.1.3.2 Class 3B lasers and laser systems include:

(1) Ultraviolet (180 to 400 nm) and infrared (1.4 μm to 1 mm) lasers and laser systems which can emit accessible radiant power in excess of the Class 3R AEL during any emission duration within the maximum duration inherent in the design of the laser or laser system, but which (a) cannot emit an average radiant power in excess of 0.5 W for $T \geq 0.25$ s or (b) cannot produce a radiant energy greater than 0.125 J within an exposure time $T < 0.25$ s.

(2) Visible (400 to 700 nm) and near-infrared (700 nm to 1.4 μm) lasers and laser systems which emit in excess of the AEL of Class 3R but which (a) cannot emit an average radiant power in excess of 0.5 W for $T \geq 0.25$ s or (b) cannot emit a radiant energy greater than 0.03 C_A J per pulse for pulses exceeding 0.5 W peak power. For this limit, all pulses within t_{min} are considered one pulse.

4.2.1.1.4 Class 4 Lasers and Laser Systems. Class 4 lasers and laser systems are those that emit radiation that exceeds the Class 3B AEL. Class 4 lasers are high power lasers that could produce skin hazards or diffuse reflection eye hazards as well as point-source viewing hazards. There is no maximum limit for Class 4 lasers.

4.3 Laser Hazard Evaluation and Hazard Class Determination.

Before measurements are undertaken, it is important that the measurement set will be useful for its intended purpose. For example, laser classification requires measurements of power or energy per pulse through specific apertures at specific distances from the laser. Appendix D provides information on laser hazard evaluation and class determination.

5. Laser Measurements

5.1 Wavelength (Spectral Content).

Often, the operating wavelength is known or specified by the laser manufacturer and does not need to be measured. The spectral content is critical, especially for lasers operating near each end of the retinal hazard region, and for lasers that can emit more than one wavelength. The spectral content of the laser radiation can be measured using commercial wavemeters, optical spectrum analyzers, monochromators, or special wavelength filters. To avoid damage to the measurement apparatus from high-power lasers, a small portion of the beam can be used to measure the wavelength.

5.2 Limiting and Measurement Apertures.

The limiting apertures for hazard evaluation and the measurement apertures for classification and assessing exposure are provided in Tables 1 and 2 of this document and in Tables 8a, 8b, and 9 of ANSI Z136.1-2007 or the most recent version. The fraction of the power or energy transmitted through various apertures is needed to evaluate biological effects on the eye and skin.

It is also necessary to know the total power or energy per pulse to perform a hazard evaluation. To properly choose the appropriate aperture(s), it may be important to measure pulse duration and repetition rate accurately. More than one measurement aperture may be needed if the values for different models are not constant over exposure times versus single pulse duration.

5.3 Power or Energy.

A radiometer is typically used to measure power or energy and provide a reading in watts or joules. The total power may be measured directly by placing a detector larger than the laser output aperture into the beam at the laser exit port. If the laser exit port is not accessible, it is necessary to know the approximate beam diameter to know how large a detector to use to collect the entire beam. If the laser beam is larger than the size of available detectors, a focusing lens can be used to reduce the beam size. If this is done, the optical losses due to lens reflection and absorption must be taken into account.

Energy per pulse may be measured directly in a similar manner or computed from peak power and pulse width. Determine the pulse width from the half-power points. The product of the peak power and pulse width approximates the area under the power vs. time curve. Instruments that can perform an integration of power vs. time will yield more accurate results.

Effective power or energy is measured similarly to total power or energy, except that the measurement is made through an applicable aperture at a particular measurement distance.

Power and energy measurements are often not as simple as merely putting a detector in front of a laser and reading the meter. For pulsed or scanning beams, the maximum repetition rate to which the energy meter will respond is provided by the manufacturer and should not be exceeded unless the results can be corrected using manufacturer-suggested guidelines. When measuring pulse energy or average power, never exceed the maximum ratings provided by the detector manufacturer. If the pulse energy saturates the detector, the reading will be lower than the actual power or energy in the beam.

The average pulse energy can also be calculated by dividing the average power by the PRF; however, many detectors do not have the dynamic range to accurately track the peak power, especially on the higher scales. If the maximum current is reached during the pulse, the reading will be low. A saturation check can be made by reducing the energy irradiating the detector by a factor (such as 10) and checking that the indication on the instrument is reduced by that same factor. If the indication of the reduced energy is higher than it should be, then saturation should be suspected.

Locating the laser beam may require infrared viewers, phosphorescent materials, thermal liquid crystal sheets, photographic film or other beam detection equipment so that measurements can be performed and it can be verified that the entire beam is in the detector.

5.4 Irradiance and Radiant Exposure.

Some instruments are designed to measure irradiance or radiant exposure directly by dividing the power or energy received by the active area of the device. Since MPEs are provided in terms of irradiance or radiant exposure, these instruments are useful for taking measurements at various exposure locations for direct comparison with the MPEs. In these situations, the laser energy will usually be spread over a large area. The detector is able to sample specific locations for potential laser exposure.

These instruments prove less useful for measuring the irradiance or radiant exposure in the direct beam of a laser. When the active area of the detector is small compared with the beam diameter, the maximum reading corresponds to the peak irradiance or peak radiant exposure in the beam. When the beam is smaller than the active area of the detector, power or energy may be calculated by multiplying the reading by the effective active area of the detector. When the beam is approximately the same size as the active area of the detector, accurate readings of any radiometric quantity are difficult to determine from the measured value of a single instrument of this kind.

5.5 Apparent Visual Angle (Angular Subtense α).

Considering a source to be a point source is a more conservative approach for sources that subtend angles larger than 1.5 mrad. An instrument that measures only the portion of energy within α_{min}, in addition to other measurements, is useful in determining ocular hazards. An instrument with an adjustable field of view is useful for assessing photochemical hazards in the wavelength band of 400-600 nm. To assess photochemical hazards (for T_{max} greater than 10 s), the field of view (FOV) should be adjusted to the limiting cone angle, γ, specified in ANSI Z136.1-2007 (11 mrad for $T_{max} \leq 100$ s).

5.5.1 Direct Viewing of an Extended Source Laser. When optics are used to expand the laser beam, reduce the divergence, or collimate the beam, the image of the source appears behind the optics and the apparent visual angle is never greater than the beam divergence. The flash distance, r_f, is the distance beyond which the magnified laser source subtends the same apparent angle as the projector lens exit port diameter. At the flash distance and greater distances, the apparent visual angle is equal to the exit aperture diameter divided by the viewing distance. That is,

$$\alpha = \frac{D_{exit}}{r_f}, \quad (1)$$

where D_{exit} is the diameter of the exit port of the laser. For nearly collimated lasers, the apparent visual angle is relatively constant from the output to the flash distance; at distances beyond the flash distance, the apparent visual angle is D_{exit}/r. Diode laser systems may have a flash distance for each dimension of the diode.

For purposes of estimation, intrabeam photographs using properly exposed infrared (or visible) film or a CCD camera, taken at several distances up to and beyond the flash distance, are helpful to account for all possible combinations of sources. Proper exposure of the film requires that the exposure be in the film's linear response region.

The apparent visual angle for a group of sources is defined by the most restrictive combination of sources. The value of α for symmetrical (or somewhat regularly shaped) sources can be obtained directly from measuring the beam size in each axis, averaging the two axis dimensions, and dividing by the viewing distance as computed from the equation,

$$\alpha = \frac{D_{Lx} + D_{Ly}}{2r_1} \quad (2)$$

An effective source size should be determined for irregular sources, which accurately describes the actual hazard. The effective apparent visual angle for any arbitrarily shaped source is defined using the average (arithmetic mean) apparent linear dimension. If one dimension is less than α_{min}, use α_{min} as that dimension. If one dimension is greater than α_{max}, eliminate the contribution of the laser emission outside of a cone equal to α_{max}, and use α_{max} as that dimension.

The source dimensions are defined in such a way that the maximum corneal irradiance (averaged over α_{min}) may be determined from dividing the total power entering the eye by the area of the beam, as defined by the assumed shape and measured dimensions. The source dimensions may be determined through imaging as shown in Figure 3.

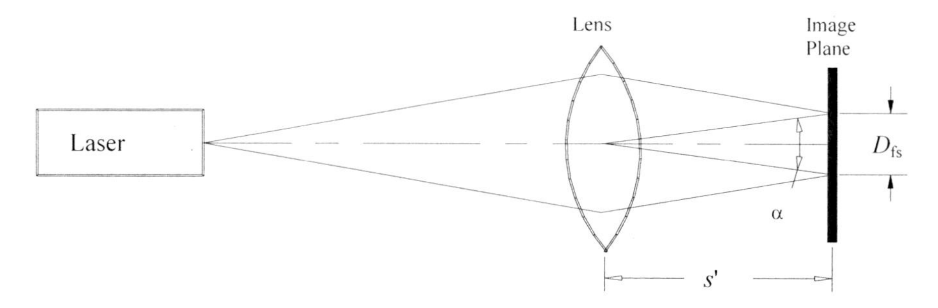

Figure 3. Illustration for Determination of Apparent Visual Angle

For sources which are basically circular but have a much higher irradiance in the center of the retinal image than in the surrounding tissue, an effective angular subtense of the source in radians may be determined by two measurements: (1) the total intraocular power in the main part of the beam, Φ_0, and (2) the maximum intraocular power, Φ_d, actually contained within a circular cone equal to α_{min}. This cone angle corresponds to the retinal area defined by a 25.5 µm diameter circle. For this estimation, the widely scattered portion of the emitted beam is not included in the total emitted power that is used in the calculation. The effective angular subtense of the source in radians can then be determined from the following formula:

$$\alpha_{eff} = \sqrt{\frac{-(0.0015)^2}{\ln\left(1 - \frac{\Phi_d}{\Phi_0}\right)}} \quad (3)$$

For example, if $\Phi_d = 0.632\ \Phi_0$, the effective angular subtense $\alpha_{eff} = \alpha_{min} = 1.5$ mrad.

5.5.2 Diffuse Laser Reflection. This type of source is produced when a laser beam strikes a diffusely reflecting surface. The apparent visual angle α is the ratio of the apparent linear dimension to the viewing distance. For example, when viewing a Gaussian beam, normal to the reflecting surface,

$$\alpha = \frac{D_L}{r_1}, \quad (4)$$

where D_L is the beam diameter at 1/e peak irradiance points on the diffuse surface and r_1 is the viewing distance.

Imaging can be used to determine α for a diffuse reflection by using the laser source to form a diffuse spot as shown in Figure 3. The equation,

$$\alpha = 2\arctan\left(\frac{D_{fs}}{2s'}\right), \quad (5)$$

where s' is the image distance and D_{fs} is the image diameter at the image plane. Imaging may be used to provide a more accurate estimate of the angular subtense for a larger diameter laser spot, such as a diffuse reflection.

When viewing a diffusely reflecting surface off axis, the angle between a normal to the diffuse surface and the viewing axis (θ_v) should be taken into account. The angular subtense in one dimension remains as calculated above, but the angular subtense in the other (orthogonal) dimension is given by

$$\alpha = \frac{D_L \cos\theta_v}{r_1} \quad (6)$$

This viewing condition is illustrated in Figure 4.

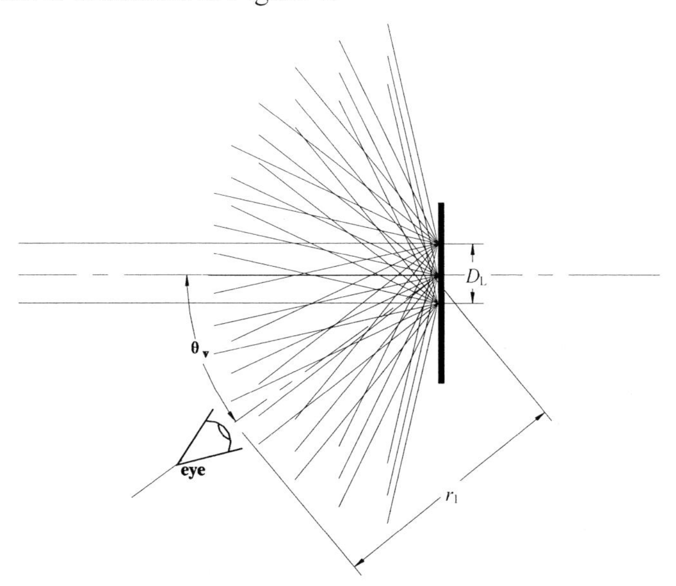

Figure 4. Diffuse Laser Reflection Viewed at Some Angle from Normal Incidence

Often θ_v is taken to be 0° (viewed perpendicular to the surface), since this is the most hazardous case. When a more detailed analysis is desired from viewing the reflected laser energy off axis, the average of the two dimensions determines the apparent visual angle for computing a C_E correction factor. Recall, if one dimension is less than α_{min}, use α_{min} as that dimension when calculating the average. When the effective apparent visual angle exceeds α_{min}, a C_E correction factor, as determined from ANSI Z136.1, may be applied to the MPE.

The irradiance or radiant exposure will also be corrected by a factor of cos θ_v. Therefore, viewing a diffuse target off axis is less hazardous than on-axis viewing; however, when the MPE and the irradiance or radiant exposure at the viewer's location are corrected based on the viewing angle, the hazard reduction is minimal when the diffuse reflection source is extended since the radiance is independent of viewing angle.

Given r_1 (see Figure 4), the value of α can be obtained directly by measuring D_L, or by calculating D_L using the propagation characteristics of the beam.

If the divergence and D_L at any point in the beam path are known, then D_L at any range can be calculated. After determining the range, the value of α can then be computed using equation (4).

5.5.3. Optical Viewing Aids. Viewing any source at a particular distance with an optical magnifier that can resolve the image of the source will multiply the apparent visual angle at that distance by the magnifying power of the magnifier.

NOTE: The radiance or integrated radiance of an extended source cannot be increased.

5.6 Beam Characteristics.

Laser safety measurements generally depend on the maximum amount of power or energy that can pass through the limiting aperture at a given range. Except for exposure to laser beams smaller than the limiting aperture, laser hazards are usually directly related to the maximum beam irradiance or radiant exposure. Thus, the beam diameter for laser safety calculations is based on 1/e peak of irradiance points rather than at $1/e^2$ points.

5.6.1 Beam Profile. Lasers can have a myriad of irradiance or radiant exposure profiles, often much different than the Gaussian, TEM_{00} mode. The center of the beam generally has the highest local irradiance value. However, hot spots in the beam can produce an increased hazard at locations in the beam other than at its center. Also, an increasing number of lasers possess an energy distribution that is approximately uniform across the entire beam.

In laser safety evaluations, beam profiles are usually modeled in one of two ways: Gaussian or uniform (sometimes called "top-hat"). Although equations using the uniform model to calculate hazard distances and eye protection requirements are much simpler, they can produce unacceptable error when dealing with lasers possessing a Gaussian or other profile when the beam dimensions are approximately the same size as the measurement aperture. In these cases, determining the proper model is important when conducting a laser hazard evaluation.

5.6.2 Beam Shape. Lasers may emit beams that are circular, rectangular, elliptical, annular, or otherwise irregular. When dealing with non-circular laser beams, the beam dimension in each axis should be determined. It is not uncommon for lasers to have different beam profiles and propagation properties in each axis. Often, it is useful to measure maximum beam irradiance or radiant exposure at different ranges from the laser, especially with irregular beam shapes and profiles.

5.6.3 Beam Size. The beam size can either be measured directly or calculated using a given beam profile model. If the divergence, ϕ, and size D_{L1} at a given point at a distance r_1 from the beam waist in the beam path are known, the beam size D_{L2} at a range r_2 beyond the beam waist can be calculated by using these equations:

$$D_{L2} = \sqrt{(r_2^2 - r_1^2) \cdot \phi^2 + D_{L1}^2} \qquad (7)$$

for the hyperbolic beam expansion model (where r_0 is the external beam waist distance, note Section 5.7), and

$$D_{L2} = (r_2 - r_1) \cdot \phi + D_{L1} \qquad (8)$$

for the linear beam expansion model. Note that units for D_{L1}, r_1, and r_2 must all be the same.

5.6.4 Direct Measurements. There are several methods for measuring beam diameter or dimensions; some are listed below.

5.6.4.1 Circular Aperture Energy Measurement. In this method, a detector measures the total radiation passing through a variable aperture. The aperture is adjusted until approximately 63.2% of the total radiation reaches the detector. The diameter of the aperture is then equal to the 1/e beam diameter if the beam were Gaussian. This method is only valid if the beam is circularly symmetric and if the aperture is centered on the beam. A small fixed aperture of diameter D_{fa} may be placed in the center of the beam to collect a fraction of the laser power or energy, represented by Φ_d/Φ_0. If the beam is assumed Gaussian or top-hat in shape, and the fraction is less than 80%, beam diameter D_L can be approximated by

$$D_L = \sqrt{\frac{-D_{fa}^2}{\ln\left(1 - \frac{\Phi_d}{\Phi_0}\right)}} \qquad (9)$$

for a Gaussian beam, and

$$D_L = D_{fa}\sqrt{\frac{\Phi_0}{\Phi_d}} \qquad (10)$$

for a top-hat shaped beam profile.

5.6.4.2 Scanning Slit Measurement. In this method a detector measures the radiation passing through a narrow slit located between the detector and the laser beam source. The detector response is monitored as the slit is scanned across the beam and the beam diameter is then the distance between the scan locations where the reading has dropped to approximately 36.8% of maximum. The accuracy of this type of measurement relies on the slit width being much smaller than the beam size. The scanning axis can be rotated to measure the beam size on different axes. For a uniform beam profile, the difference in positions on each side of the beam where the laser beam energy declines rapidly is the beam diameter. The scanning slit technique is often used on commercial beam profile systems. The use of unguarded razor blades for this operation is not recommended.

5.6.4.3 Scanning Knife Edge. This method is similar in principal to the scanning slit method except that a single knife edge is used instead of a slit. The output of the detector is then related to the integral (along one axis) of the irradiance distribution. Assuming a Gaussian beam profile, the knife edge is positioned at the location where 86.5% of the energy is transmitted to the detector and at the location where 13.5% of the energy is transmitted to the detector. The difference in these two positions provides the $1/e^2$ beam radius. As with the scanning slit, for a uniform beam profile, the difference in positions on each side of the beam where the laser beam energy begins to decline and where the beam energy is barely detectable, is the beam diameter. Once the $1/e^2$ beam diameter is found, it can be converted to the 1/e beam diameter by dividing the $1/e^2$ beam diameter by $\sqrt{2}$. The use of unguarded razor blades for this operation is not recommended.

5.6.4.4 Pinhole Aperture. In this method, the output of a detector is monitored as a pinhole aperture (placed between the detector and the laser beam) is scanned across the two-dimensional plane of the laser beam. This method is simple in principle but inherently takes more time to accomplish and thus relies on stable laser output during the measurement period. The beam diameter is then defined as the average radial distance between two points where the local beam irradiance drops to 1/e (i.e., 37%) times the center beam irradiance. This technique may not be appropriate for small beams.

5.6.4.5 CCD Camera or Pyroelectric Array. In this method, the entire beam is sampled at one time using a two dimensional array of optically sensitive elements. In concept, it is similar to the pinhole method because it measures the entire beam profile at one plane location. This method is used when the irradiance profile of the entire beam is needed or when high resolution is required. Commercial instruments using this concept are commonly available.

5.6.4.6 Visual Observations. The beam diameter can be estimated by measuring or estimating the visual size of (1) scattered or emitted radiation from materials (such as fluorescent cards, colored paper, etc.) placed in the beam or (2) burn/exposure patterns produced on a target (such as acrylic plastic, thermal paper, tongue depressors, photographic film, etc.). This method is often deceptive since the apparent size of the beam changes depending on ambient illumination, the power of the laser beam, and properties of the absorbing and reflecting surface. This method should be used with caution and is not recommended for quantitative assessment.

5.7 Beam Waist.

It is possible for a laser to have an external beam waist, which will increase the hazard distance. The location of the beam waist can often be found easily within the first few meters of the exit port of the laser by measuring the beam diameter at several points from the output until it is clear that the beam is expanding. If the beam diameter at some range away from the laser is found to be smaller than the exit beam diameter, then the smallest diameter found is the external beam waist diameter D_W, and the distance from the laser to the waist is r_0. The following equation then applies for the beam diameter at a range r from the laser:

$$D_L = \sqrt{D_W^2 + (r - r_0)^2 \cdot \phi^2} \qquad (11)$$

The equation for calculating beam diameter for laser safety does not assume any particular mode of operation for the laser. For lasers with no external beam waist, D_W is the exit beam diameter, and r_0 is eliminated from the above equation. Since no particular operating mode is assumed, the value of D_W cannot be used to determine the beam divergence. The beam divergence can be determined by the techniques in the next Section (5.8). It is possible for non-circular beams to have a beam waist in each dimension at different distances, requiring special consideration.

5.8 Beam Divergence.

There are several ways to determine beam divergence; some are listed below.

5.8.1 Two-point Diameter Measurement. The beam divergence can be found by knowing the beam diameter at the beam waist and another point in the laser beam as provided in the following equation:

$$\phi = \frac{\sqrt{D_L^2 - D_W^2}}{(r - r_0)} \qquad (12)$$

Once the waist diameter and location are determined, a measurement of the beam size at some range where the beam has expanded substantially (at least fifty percent) can be used to determine the beam divergence. Caution must be used to ensure measurements are made in the far field. Two independent measurements can be done at various ranges using the two-point method to ensure agreement with increasing range.

Another method is to choose two points along the beam path where the beam diameter is substantially larger than the beam waist (see Figure 5). The following equation will then provide a simpler expression for beam divergence, where D_{L1} and D_{L2} are beam diameter measurements, and $r_{2\text{-}1}$ is the distance separating the two measurement positions.

$$\phi = \frac{D_{L2} - D_{L1}}{r_{2-1}} \qquad (13)$$

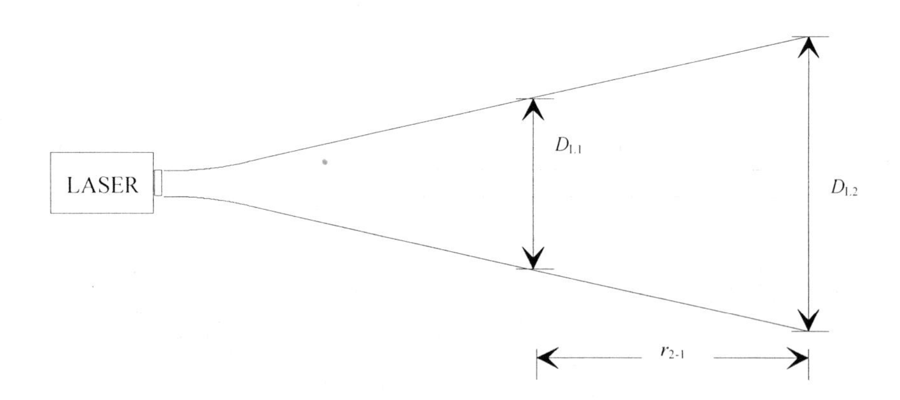

Figure 5. Two-Point Beam Diameter Measurement

5.8.2 Long Focal Length Lens and Aperture Technique. If a long focal length lens is used to focus the laser beam, the diameter of the beam at the focal plane can be used to determine the beam divergence (see Figure 6). The small aperture is used to measure the beam diameter of the laser beam at the focal point of the lens. The location of the lens in front of the laser is not critical, but the lens should not be placed at the beam waist.

The geometric focal length of the lens at the particular laser wavelength should be determined, if not known in advance or specified by the manufacturer. A lamp may be used to determine the focal length, according to the following formula,

$$\frac{1}{s_1}+\frac{1}{s_2}=\frac{1}{f}, \tag{14}$$

where s_1 is the distance from the lens to the image and s_2 is the distance from the lens to the object. If the lamp is placed at about twice the focal length, the image will appear at about twice the focal length on the other side. The formula above may then be used to determine the geometric focal length, by measuring the location of the image. A narrow pass filter may be used to measure the focal length of the lens for various laser wavelengths.

The beam divergence from a laser is determined from the beam diameter at the geometrical focal point (or infinity focal point) D_{fp} of this lens,

$$\phi=\frac{D_{\mathrm{fp}}}{f} \tag{15}$$

The beam diameter at the focal plane is not necessarily the smallest beam diameter. A beam waist located between the lens and the measuring aperture is an indication of an external beam waist beyond the lens position.

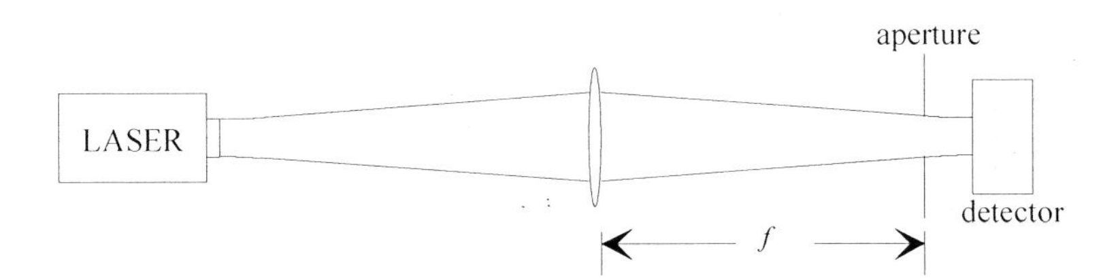

Figure 6. Arrangement for Long Focal Length Lens and Small Aperture

5.8.3 Irradiance Measurement. Beam divergence may be determined from the total power output Φ and a single, maximized irradiance measurement E_{max} in the center of the beam at some distance from the laser. The area of the detector should be significantly smaller than the beam diameter at the place of measurement. At a distance r from the laser, where the initial beam diameter is negligible, the divergence for a Gaussian profile-shape beam may be calculated from

$$\phi = \frac{\sqrt{\frac{4\Phi}{\pi E_{max}}}}{r} \quad (16)$$

5.9 Pulse Characteristics.

In addition to CW operation, laser radiation may be emitted in a single pulse or in repetitive pulses. Generally, the temporal characteristics are available from the manufacturer. When it is necessary to characterize the time-varying output, a detector with a time constant of at least ten times shorter than pulse rise time should be used. Measurements include PRF and pulse duration.

5.9.1 Pulse Duration (Δt). To measure pulse duration, expose a fast detector to the laser beam and observe the detector output as a function of time. The pulse width is found by measuring the time duration between the leading and trailing half power points of the pulse. For scanning CW lasers, an effective pulse duration can be found by measuring or calculating the time it takes for a beam to cross the limiting aperture.

5.9.2 Measuring the Number of Pulses in an Exposure. The number of pulses delivered during an exposure of a repetitively pulsed laser is important when determining its associated MPE. Pulse counting is usually done with a detector and either an oscilloscope or a frequency counter. When dealing with a laser that produces evenly spaced pulses, the number of pulses delivered in the exposure is simply the product of the pulse repetition rate and the exposure time.

Determining pulses that are not uniformly spaced requires careful triggering of the oscilloscope to look at a single trace instead of overlapped traces. An overlapping trace image can suggest a pulse count that is too high. The effect of counting a larger number of pulses will result in an erroneous MPE.

5.10 M-Squared (M^2).

M^2 (also called Beam Quality, Beam Propagation Ratio, or Times Diffraction limit number) is an indication of how close the energy distribution in a laser beam is to that of a perfect Gaussian beam. The diffraction-limited divergence (1/e) of a Gaussian beam is given by

$$\phi = \frac{2\lambda}{\pi D_W} \tag{17}$$

The diameter-divergence product for any beam propagating through a non-aberrating optical system (e.g., a vacuum) is constant. M^2 of a laser beam is determined by

1) measuring the waist diameter and the divergence
2) calculating the diameter-divergence product
3) dividing this value by the diameter-divergence product of a Gaussian beam of the same wavelength.

The equation relating M^2 to the divergence, beam waist diameter, and wavelength is given by

$$M^2 = \frac{\phi \pi D_W}{2\lambda} \tag{18}$$

Many laser manufacturers specify laser beams by providing M^2 and either beam diameter or divergence. For a perfect Gaussian beam $M^2 = 1$. High power multimode lasers may have an M^2 of 15 or more.

While M^2 is simple in theory, measurement can be complex for some laser beams. Numerous technical papers have documented various techniques for M^2 measurements and a careful review of such techniques and applicable optics/beam propagation theory may be required to obtain an accurate M^2 measurement.

An M^2 value is important for laser hazard calculations as the beam diameter, $D(z)$ (of a less than ideal Gaussian beam) as a function of distance, z, from the beam waist can be determined from the following equation:

$$D(z) = D_W \sqrt{1 + \frac{(z - z_0)^2}{z_R^2}} \tag{19}$$

Where D_W is the beam waist diameter, and z_0 is the beam waist position. z_R is the Rayleigh range and can be calculated as follows:

$$z_R = \frac{\pi D_W^2}{M^2 2\lambda} \tag{20}$$

These equations are useful for determining exposure vs. range and thus NOHD for a less than ideal Gaussian beam.

Appendix A
Acronyms, Abbreviations, and Variable Symbols

A1. Acronyms and Abbreviations.

AEL Accessible Emission Limit

ANSI American National Standards Institute

CW Continuous Wave

CCD Charge Coupled Device

D* Normalized Detectivity

FIR Far Infrared

FLPPS Federal Laser Product Performance Standard

FOV Field of View

FWHM Full Width Half Maximum

IEC International Electrotechnical Commission

IR Infrared

ISO International Organization for Standardization

LED Light Emitting Diode

LSO Laser Safety Officer

MPE Maximum Permissible Exposure

NEP Noise Equivalent Power

NHZ Nominal Hazard Zone

NIR Near Infrared

NOHD Nominal Ocular Hazard Distance

NSHD Nominal Skin Hazard Distance

PRF Pulse Repetition Frequency

SNR Signal to Noise Ratio

TEM Transverse Electromagnetic

UV Ultraviolet

A2. Variable Symbols.

A = Area (cm^2)

B = Bandwidth (nm)

D = Diameter (cm)

D_c = Collecting Aperture Diameter of an Optical System (cm)

D_e = Exit Diameter of Optical Aids (cm)

D_{exit} = Laser Exit Port Diameter (cm)

D_f = Limiting Aperture Diameter (cm)

D_{fa} = Small Fixed Aperture Diameter (cm)

D_{fp} = Beam Diameter at the Focal Point of a Lens (cm)

D_{fs} = Image Diameter at Image Plane (cm)

D_L = Laser Beam Diameter at Any Range (cm)

D_λ = Optical Density

D_m = Measurement Aperture Diameter (cm)

D_w = Diameter of a Beam Waist which occurs in Front of the Exit Port (cm)

E = Irradiance ($W \cdot cm^{-2}$)

f = Focal Length (cm)

H = Radiant Exposure ($J \cdot cm^{-2}$)

I = Radiant Intensity, Input

L = Radiance ($W \cdot cm^{-2} \cdot sr^{-1}$)

M = Magnification of Optics

O = Output

P_s = Optical Signal Power

r = Range (cm)

R = Responsivity

s = Distance (cm)

t = Time, Duration (s)

T = Exposure Duration(s)

Q = Energy (J)

α = Angular Subtense (mrad)

γ = Limiting Cone Angle (mrad)

λ = Wavelength (μm)

μ = Attenuation (cm^{-1})

Ω = Solid Angle (sr)

ϕ = Divergence (mrad)

Φ = Radiant Power (W)

θ = Angle of Incidence

τ = Transmittance

A3. Photobiological Quantities.

For all photobiological effects, it is necessary to measure the appropriate radiometric quantity. The surface exposure dose rate is termed the *irradiance,* with units of watts per square centimeter ($W \cdot cm^{-2}$), and the surface exposure dose is termed the *radiant exposure,* with units of joules per square centimeter ($J \cdot cm^{-2}$). There are also parallel dose rate and dose concepts within scattering tissue, and these quantities are termed *fluence rate,* also with units of watts per square centimeter ($W \cdot cm^{-2}$), and dose within tissue that is termed the *fluence,* also with units of joules per square centimeter ($J \cdot cm^{-2}$). The existence of two terms for the same radiometric unit seems curious, and this has confused many scientists, with the result that the terms are frequently misused. But the concepts are different and the distinctions are important. The quantities irradiance and radiant exposure are what instruments measure at the exposed surface (and follow Lambert's Cosine Law), but fluence rate and fluence include backscattered light and are useful for photochemical calculations within tissue (as in photodynamic therapy). Table A1 provides the principal current internationally standardized radiometric terms and units.

Table A1. Useful Standardized International CIE Radiometric Units 1, 2

Term	Symbol	Definition	Unit and Abbreviation
Radiant Energy	Q	Energy emitted, transferred, or received in the form of radiation	joule (J)
Radiant Power	Φ	Radiant Energy per unit time	watt (W) defined as $J \cdot s^{-1}$
Radiant Exposure (Dose in Photobiology)	H	Energy per unit area incident upon a given surface	joules per square centimeter ($J \cdot cm^{-2}$)
Irradiance or Radiant Flux Density (Dose Rate in Photobiology)	E	Power per unit area incident upon a given surface	watts per square centimeter ($W \cdot cm^{-2}$)
Integrated Radiant Intensity	I_P	Radiant Energy emitted by a source per unit solid angle	joules per steradian ($J \cdot sr^{-1}$)
Radiant Intensity	I	Radiant Power emitted by a source per unit solid angle	watts per steradian ($W \cdot sr^{-1}$)
Integrated Radiance	L_P	Radiant Energy emitted by a source per unit solid angle per unit source area	joules per steradian per square centimeter ($J \cdot sr^{-1} \cdot cm^{-2}$)
Radiance[3]	L	Radiant Power emitted by a source per unit solid angle per unit source area	watts per steradian per square centimeter ($W \cdot sr^{-1} \cdot cm^{-2}$)
Optical Density	OD	A logarithmic expression for the attenuation produced by a medium $OD = -\log_{10}\left(\frac{\Phi_\tau}{\Phi_i}\right)$	unitless Φ_i is the incident power; Φ_τ is the transmitted power

1. The units may be altered to refer to narrow spectral bands in which the term is preceded by the word *spectral* and the unit is then per wavelength interval and the symbol has a subscript λ. For example, spectral irradiance E_λ has units of $W \cdot m^{-2} \cdot m^{-1}$ or more often, $W \cdot cm^{-2} \cdot nm^{-1}$.

2. While the meter is the preferred unit of length, the centimeter is still the most commonly used unit of length for many of the terms above and the nm or μm are most commonly used to express wavelength.

3. At the source $L = \dfrac{dI}{dA \cdot \cos\theta}$ and at a receptor $L = \dfrac{dE}{d\Omega \cdot \cos\theta}$.

Appendix B
Detectors

B1. Thermal Detectors.

Thermal detectors absorb laser radiation and convert the electromagnetic energy to thermal energy. The change in thermal energy results in a temperature change which is correlated to the input power of the laser radiation. To capture the laser energy, thermal detectors frequently use coatings of highly absorbent materials, such as black paint or a gold-black metal layer, whose photon absorbing properties typically do not vary significantly over broad wavelength ranges. Consequently, for a given incident power, the responsivity of a thermal detector is usually relatively constant or *flat* over a wide wavelength region. Due to their inherent structure and mode of operation, thermal detectors are usually slower than quantum detectors but can accommodate higher powers. Some thermal detectors can be calibrated electrically with built-in electrical heaters.

B.1.1 Thermopile-based Detectors. A thermopile-based detector uses one or more thermocouples electrically connected in series and placed in thermal contact to a laser radiation absorbing material such as a coated metal disc. Thermocouples produce a voltage, by a mechanism known as the Seebeck effect, proportional to the temperature difference at the junction of two dissimilar materials. Since the temperature change of the absorbing material is proportional to the absorbed laser energy, the electrical output of the thermopile can be used as a measure of the incident laser power.

In general, the range and sensitivity of the thermopile detector are a result of the thermal properties of the thermopile and the radiation absorber to which it is attached. Thermopile detectors for high power or energy and fast response times are typically designed to quickly dissipate most of the heat absorbed by the detector. When a detector is designed to have an inefficient heat path away from the absorption structure, the instrument acts as an energy storage device and is relatively slow to reach steady state. This slower type of device is often used to measure energy and is called a "calorimeter," whereas the device with faster heat flow is generally called a "power meter."

B.1.2 Bolometer. A bolometer is a detector that primarily consists of a temperature sensitive electrical resistor. The resistor impedance is a direct function of temperature which, in turn, is proportional to absorbed laser power or energy. A bolometer is usually operated in a bridge circuit with the sensing resistor element exposed to laser radiation and with a compensating element exposed to reference conditions (ambient conditions or an electrical equivalent). A thermistor-based detector is similar, but features a metal oxide or semiconductor resistive element, in which the relationship between resistance and temperature is not necessarily linear.

B.1.3 Pyroelectric-based Detectors. Pyroelectric-based detectors are made using a pyroelectric material (an electret) sandwiched between two electrodes and coated with an absorbing material such as black paint. The radiation absorbed by the absorbing material is converted into heat, which raises the temperature of the electret. This change in temperature alters the lattice spacing of the pyroelectric material and produces a change in the spontaneous polarization in the material. An electrical current is generated to balance the polarization change, which is proportional to the rate of change of temperature of the electret. The current generated can be converted to a voltage which is proportional to incident laser power.

Pyroelectric detectors respond only to pulsed, modulated, or chopped radiation sources. A continuous source laser beam can be measured but is normally chopped mechanically. As with other thermal detectors, these detectors exhibit a broad spectral response that is limited by the characteristics of the absorbing material and the transmittance of any window. Small area pyroelectric detectors also exhibit fast response times (1 ns) and are the most sensitive of the thermal detectors. Pyroelectric detectors are sometimes used in an electrical substitution scheme with an electrical heater attached to the detector. This type of pyroelectric is called an electrically calibrated pyroelectric radiometer or ECPR.

B2. Quantum Detectors.

Quantum detectors respond electrically upon absorption of individual photons, but the nature of this response varies for different materials and material structures. Most quantum detectors are made of semiconductor materials, but photographic emulsions can also be considered as quantum detectors, since individual quanta are absorbed by silver halides and a latent image is the result of a photochemical process. Photographic detectors measure total photon exposure or energy. Although not widely used for evaluation of laser hazards because of slow speed, limited spectral responsivity, and nonlinear responsivity, they are sometimes used to measure the approximate source size. Photoluminescent materials are also quantum detectors and are typically used for laser alignment, but not used to measure power and energy.

B.2.1 Photoemitter-based Detectors. Photoemitter-based detectors use the photoelectric effect in which a photocathode surface is struck by incoming photons and emits electrons. These electrons are accelerated across an electric potential difference and collected at an anode while generating a current in an external circuit. These detectors must therefore have an external power supply. Photoemissive detectors are relatively sensitive and can be used at short wavelengths, but may have poor spatial uniformity and may require more frequent calibration.

Vacuum phototubes consist of a photocathode and an anode enclosed in a sealed tube and connected in series with a resistor and a voltage supply. The voltage drop across the resistor is proportional to the photon-generated current when photons are incident on the photocathode. Such biplanar phototubes are suitable for pulsed laser measurements with less than 1 ns rise times.

Photomultipliers are photoemissive detectors that operate on the same principle as the phototube except that secondary surfaces, called dynodes, amplify the current by as much as 6 orders of magnitude. These detectors are fast with rise times of about 3 ns but require very stable, high voltage power supplies for reliable measurements.

B.2.2 Semiconductor Detectors.

B.2.2.1 Photoconductor-based Detectors. Photoconductors are quantum detectors that consist of a homogeneous semiconductor material. Photons incident on the material are absorbed and create additional free electrons that lower the material resistance or increase the current in the presence of an external bias. An external power supply is necessary, but the detector can be biased in either direction. Current through or voltage across a fixed series resistance are normally the measured electrical quantities for photoconductors, and these detectors are often cryogenically cooled to improve detectivity over a broader wavelength range. In general, these detectors are slower (1-ms response time) than other quantum detectors but exhibit high detectivities in the mid to far IR.

B.2.2.2 Photovoltaic-based Detectors. Photovoltaic detectors are PN junction photodiodes consisting of a positively-doped P region and a negatively-doped N region with a depletion region of neutral charge in between. To improve the performance of the device, one type of photodiode, called a PIN photodiode has an intrinsic (I) or pure semiconductor layer in the junction that widens the depletion region. Incident photons of energy greater than or equal to the energy band gap of the semiconductor material generate electron-hole pairs or charge carriers. Electron-hole pairs generated in the depletion region are separated by the junction electric field and drift to the oppositely charged electrodes of the detector and produce a current through an external circuit or instrument. When the circuit is properly designed, the measured current is proportional to the incident optical power. The semiconductor photodiode can be used with either zero or reverse bias. Reverse bias improves response linearity and increases the speed by lowering the junction capacitance.

A common type of photovoltaic detector is the solar cell (PN silicon). These devices have their greatest sensitivity in the visible and near infrared and exhibit about 1-μs response times but are not commonly used for quantitative measurements because of their nonlinear electrical behavior. PIN semiconductor detectors used with a bias exhibit 1-ns rise times, and about a 50% increase in sensitivity with respect to the photovoltaic mode. A silicon photodiode operated with a reverse bias is capable of peak responsivity of 0.5 A/W at a wavelength of 650 nm and is well suited for visible and near infrared (NIR) wavelength laser irradiance measurements less than 10 $mW \cdot cm^{-2}$. UV enhanced photodiodes may be used for wavelengths down to 190 nm or even lower.

Avalanche photodiodes are photodiodes fabricated to function in the presence of a relatively high external reverse-bias. Operating in the avalanche region, incident photons generate charge carriers which are accelerated by the high bias and generate secondary charge carriers, which may generate even more charge carriers.

Avalanche photodiodes are not frequently used in applications requiring high precision or accuracy because they typically have a small area, and above a certain irradiance threshold, the voltage response is independent of the number of incident photons. However, reverse-bias photodiodes operated in the avalanche region typically have a factor of 100 times increase in responsivity and a decrease in rise time from approximately 1 μs to 0.5 ns. In this mode they are most often used for high speed (short laser pulse) measurements.

Appendix C
Detector Specifications

C1. Detectors and Detector Capability Ranges for Continuous Laser Input Conditions.

[Adapted from Bass M. Optical Society of America, *Handbook of Optics, Vol. I*, McGraw Hill, Inc., New York, 1995, Budde W. *Optical Radiation Measurements, Volume 4, Physical Detectors of Optical Radiation*, Academic Press, New York, 1983, and vendor literature.]

Detector type	Wavelength (μm) range	Max Input ($W \cdot cm^{-2}$)	Response time (s)	Max Area (mm^2)	Uniformity (% spatial response variation)
Avalanche diode	0.25 - 1.9	2×10^{-4}	8×10^{-11} - 5×10^{-9}	0.007 - 7	5
Germanium photodiode	0.4 - 1.9	2×10^{-3} - 0.3	5×10^{-10} - 2×10^{-7}	0.01 - 80	5
Silicon photodiode, biased	0.25 - 1.1	5×10^{-3} - 1×10^{-2}	3×10^{-11} - 2×10^{-7}	0.01 - 800	2
Silicon photodiode, unbiased	0.25 - 1.1	5×10^{-3} - 1×10^{-2}	8×10^{-9} - 2×10^{-6}	0.85 - 800	2
Photoconductor for shorter or "near" infrared wavelengths (InSb, PbS, PbSe)	0.35 – 6	2×10^{-3}	1×10^{-6} - 5×10^{-4}	3 - 100	5
Photoconductor for longer infrared wavelengths cooled (HgCdTe)	5 – 20	1×10^{-3}	1×10^{-8} - 1×10^{-7}	0.1 - 10	10
VIS photoconductor (CdS, CdSe)	0.35 - 0.85	1×10^{-1}	2×10^{-6} - 6	20 - 500	10
Photoemissive microchannel plate	0.3 - 0.9	1×10^{-10} - 1×10^{-7}	3×10^{-10}	120 - 500	10
Photomultiplier: S-4	0.18 - 0.95	1×10^{-10}	5×10^{-10} - 2×10^{-8}	14 - 12000	20-50
Photomultiplier: S-1	0.3 - 1.1	1×10^{-7}	1.5×10^{-9} - 3.5×10^{-9}	80 - 280	20-50

Detector type	Wavelength (μm) range	Max Input ($W \cdot cm^{-2}$)	Response time (s)	Max Area (mm^2)	Uniformity (% spatial response variation)
Vacuum phototube, high bias voltage	0.2 - 1.1	2×10^{-8} - 2×10^{-4}	1×10^{-10} - 1×10^{-9}	78 - 18000	20-50
Vacuum phototube, low bias voltage	0.2 - 1.1	1×10^{-3}	5×10^{-10} - 1×10^{-8}	25 - 7000	20 - 50
Pyroelectric detectors	0.2 - 25	2×10^{-1} - 10	1×10^{-9} - 1×10^{-7}	1 - 1000	5
Bolometers and Thermistors	0.2 - 25	200 - 1000	1×10^{-3}	0.01 - 100	10
Thermopile-based	0.2 - 20	50 - 5000	1×10^{-3} - 1	100 - 2000	5 - 10

C2. Detectors and Detector Capability Ranges for Pulsed Laser Input Conditions.

[Adapted from Bass M. Optical Society of America, *Handbook of Optics, Vol. I*, McGraw Hill, Inc., New York, 1995, Budde W. *Optical Radiation Measurements, Volume 4, Physical Detectors of Optical Radiation*, Academic Press, New York, 1983, and vendor literature.]

Detector type	Wavelength (μm) range	Max Input ($J \cdot cm^{-2}$) range (duration < 1 s)	Max Single Pulse Energy (J)	Max Area (mm^2)
Germanium photodiode	0.4 - 1.9	50×10^{-6} - 500×10^{-6}	50×10^{-6} - 500×10^{-6}	0.01 - 80
Silicon photodiode	0.25 - 1.1	50×10^{-6} - 1×10^{-3}	50×10^{-6} - 1×10^{-3}	0.01 - 800
Pyroelectric detector	0.2 - 25	8 - 80	1×10^{-6} - 10×10^{-3}	1 - 1000
Thermopile, surface	0.2 - 20	0.1 - 100	0.001 - 0.15	0.8 - 70
Thermopile, volume	0.2 - 20	0.5 - 1000	0.1×10^{-3} - 100	100 - 2000

Appendix D
Laser Hazard Evaluation and Classification

D1. General.

Measurements intended to be used to evaluate laser hazards require that the measurements be performed in a specific manner to simulate actual exposure to a laser beam. Hazard classification makes no assumptions on actual exposure, but establishes the hazard potential of a laser under a variety of viewing conditions based on specific test methods. A complete hazard evaluation or hazard classification requires that the following beam parameters be determined.

D2. Wavelength or Wavelengths.

Single wavelengths can be measured using a spectrometer or spectrograph. Common wavelengths are specified and may not need to be measured. If the laser emits multiple wavelengths, the hazard evaluation process becomes more complex. The average power or the energy per pulse at each wavelength is used to determine the additive effects. For a given biological exposure site (corneal, retinal or skin), the effects from each exposure condition are additive. For more information, see Terry L. Lyon, "Hazard Analysis Technique for Multiple Wavelength Lasers", *Health Physics*, Vol. 49, No. 2 (August), pp.221-226, 1985.

D3. Pulse Properties (Temporal Profile).

The inherent design of the laser determines if the laser is pulsed or CW. If the laser is pulsed, the determination of pulse width, pulse repetition frequency and/or structure of pulse groups is necessary. Pulse duration is measured at FWHM or other specification which provides average power during the pulse. Some lasers thought to be CW may in fact have a pulse structure more rapid than is visually perceptible.

D4. Exposure Duration (T).

The exposure duration may change for various exposure scenarios and applications. Each of these scenarios may need to be evaluated independently. T_{max} is the maximum exposure duration which is specifically limited by the design or intended use(s) of the laser or laser system. For classification, T_{max} can be assumed to be up to 30,000 s for 180-700 cm and 100 s for 700 nm - 1.0 mm, if the application is unknown. For example, a person in an airplane that flies through a laser beam may be exposed for only a few milliseconds, but would usually be exposed to at least one entire Q-switched pulse. For a Q-switched, repetitively pulsed laser, it is important to determine the maximum number of laser pulses during the exposure interval. For repetitive-pulsed lasers in the retinal hazard region, see ANSI Z136.1-2007 Section 8.2.3.2.

D5. Beam Diameter (D_L) and Divergence (ϕ).

Beam diameter and divergence are critical values for determining the irradiance or radiant exposure at a distance from the laser. The beam divergence and the beam diameter are usually determined at 1/e peak irradiance points for purposes of hazard evaluation. For a circular laser beam operating in the Gaussian TEM_{00} mode, the diameter of the portion of the beam which contains 63.2% of the total power or energy per pulse is considered the beam diameter for safety calculations. Note that the beam diameter and beam divergence for TEM_{00} mode Gaussian beams are 0.707 times their respective values at the $1/e^2$ irradiance points. See Sections 5.6 and 5.8 for methods of determining beam diameter and beam divergence. For elliptical, rectangular or non-Gaussian beams, methods for computing the irradiance or radiant exposure averaged over the limiting aperture as a function of distance from the laser must be devised.

D6. Angular Subtense (Angular Source Size or Apparent Visual Angle).

Also see Sec. 5.5. When a laser could illuminate a discernable area of the retina (e.g., larger than a point source), it is said to be an extended source. The MPE can be relaxed when this occurs. To determine the degree to which the MPE can be relaxed, it is necessary to determine the angular subtense from the laser. This value is a function of range and therefore can significantly increase the difficulty of hazard evaluation and classification.

If the beam is axis-symmetric there is one value for the angular subtense at a given distance; however, for non-axis-symmetric beams there may be more than one value for the angular subtense. The angular subtense for extended source lasers will be larger than α_{min} (1.5 mrad) in either dimension near the laser exit port, but is generally inversely proportional to the beam diameter at farther viewing distances. Beyond the distance where the exit aperture, D_{exit}, of the laser appears filled with laser energy (from an intrabeam point of view), the angular source size is limited by that aperture (source size would be equal to the exit aperture divided by the viewing distance). If the NOHD is farther than a few meters, the laser will generally be considered a point source at the NOHD.

For sources with divergences less than 1.5 mrad, angular subtense does not need to be determined for unaided viewing conditions, since there is no correction for source size in this AEL calculation.

D7. Total Power or Energy.

The total power or energy must be determined for hazard evaluation. The formulas used to compute irradiance or radiant exposure at a distance require the total laser power or pulse energy, the beam diameter and beam divergence. The hazards at each distance are computed from the portion of the power or energy transmitted through the measurement aperture.

D8. MPE.

The MPE for the eye can be determined from Tables 5a and 5b of ANSI Z136.1-2007. Table 5a is used for point-source lasers. For wavelengths less than 600 nm, the MPE is determined based on both photochemical and thermal effects. The thermal MPE for the eye for a source size larger than 1.5 mrad is corrected by a factor, C_E (see Section 3.2.3.4.2 and Table 5b of ANSI Z136.1-2007.) The MPE for skin exposure is provided in Table 7 of ANSI Z136.1-2007. Additional information is available in Sections 8 and 9 of ANSI Z136.1-2007.

Evaluation of pulsed exposure can be summed up in three rules: (1) The exposure from any single pulse in a train of pulses shall not exceed the MPE for a single pulse of that duration, $\boldsymbol{t}$; (2) the summed exposure from any group of pulses within a duration, $\boldsymbol{T}$, shall not exceed the MPE for a single pulse of that duration $\boldsymbol{T}$; (3) the exposure from a number of pulses, $\boldsymbol{n}$, shall not exceed the MPE for a single pulse multiplied by a factor, $\boldsymbol{C_P}$, based on $\boldsymbol{n}^{-0.25}$. The last rule applies only to ocular exposure. Also, for this rule, when the PRF is high enough that the interpulse spacing is less than t_{min} (termed the critical frequency), groups or trains of pulses are treated as a single pulse and quantified with the energy of the entire group or train. Above the critical frequency, the average power generally determines the hazards of a laser rather than exposure to individual pulses. Determination of critical frequency must be modified for extended exposure times, for extended source lasers and for sub-nanosecond pulses. Additionally, critical frequency for wavelengths outside the retinal hazard region may vary as a function of beam size.

For extended sources, the MPE for optically aided viewing is different from that for unaided viewing. In the retinal hazard region, the angular source size at the measurement distance is multiplied by the magnifying power of the optical instrument. It is important to realize that source size decreases with distance from the laser and may be reduced at the minimum distance of 2 m from what it was at 10 cm. For the binoculars recommended in hazard classification, the magnifying power is 7. However, other optical instruments may have a magnifying power of 10, 20, or more. For example, a small-beam laser source subtending an angle of 0.5 mrad at a viewing distance of 10 meters would appear to subtend an angle of 3.5 mrad for 7×50 binocular viewing at that same range, resulting in a relaxed (larger) MPE than for unaided viewing. Measurement of source size may not be necessary as assuming the laser to be a point source will provide a worst-case analysis.

D9. Limiting Aperture (D_f).

Table 1 (Tables 8a and 8b of ANSI Z136.1-2007) list the appropriate limiting apertures for the eye and skin, which depend on wavelength and exposure duration. Useful highlights from ANSI Z136.1-2007, are repeated and given in more detail in Table 1. The limiting aperture for the eye from Table 1 of this document is the same for unaided and optically aided viewing conditions. The corneal irradiance or corneal radiant exposure is averaged over the limiting aperture when compared with the MPE for hazard evaluation. When repeated exposures are evaluated using rule 1, the limiting aperture is determined by the pulse width. When the MPE is evaluated using rule 3, the exposure duration, $\boldsymbol{t}$, and associated limiting aperture is minimally limited to T_{max}. When the laser is evaluated using rules 2 and 3, the exposure duration of each pulse grouping and also T_{max} may require measurements through several aperture diameters.

D10. Measurement Aperture.

Table 2 (Table 9 from ANSI Z136.1-2007) can be used to determine the measurement aperture(s). For ocular hazards, different apertures are needed for optically aided viewing and unaided viewing (Conditions 1 and 2). When the laser operates in a wavelength region not transmitted by common optics, the measurement aperture is the same as the limiting aperture for the eye. The measurement aperture for skin hazards is the same as the skin limiting aperture. Note that, when performing evaluations on repetitive pulsed lasers, the measurement aperture for each rule may be different because of the time base used for each model.

D11. Laser Hazard Class.

Commercial lasers are classified and labeled by the manufacturer, and the user may be able to use this information to determine the class for the purposes of hazard evaluation. It is important to note that the FLPPS product classification may be different from ANSI classification. ANSI classification does not change the FLPPS product classification, so the original laser product is still subject to the same built-in control measures. Classification provides a quick assessment of the hazard potential of a particular laser.

To determine the appropriate ANSI laser hazard class, the following steps may be used:

D.11.1 Assume Laser Class. Perform a quick check of laser parameters and compare the output to the known AEL values. For example, a small beam laser with an average output power of 500 W would certainly be a Class 4 laser.

D.11.2 Measurement Distance. Measurement distances are given in Table 2. The measurement distance should not be less than 10 cm from the apparent source for unaided viewing and not less than 2 m from the laser exit port for optically aided viewing (condition 1), due to the inability of the eye or binocular to focus at shorter distances.

D.11.3 AELs. Classification is based on eye hazards, not skin hazards. The Class 1 AEL is the product of the MPE for the eye and the area of the limiting aperture for the eye. For repetitive pulses or pulse groups, several sets of measurements through various aperture diameters may be required to determine the most restrictive exposure condition. Refer to Section 4.2.1 for discussion of AELs for other classes.

D.11.4 Effective Power or Pulse Energy. Classification is based on the effective power or energy rather than the total power or energy. Effective power or pulse energy measurements are required at the appropriate distance through the appropriate aperture. Typically for a CW laser, the highest power observed over T_{max} is used for hazard classification. For repetitively pulsed lasers with fairly uniform pulse energies and pulse widths, the average energy per pulse may be measured. See Figure D-1 for additional information. Note that the measurement apertures used to determine effective power or energy may depend on the applicable viewing condition.

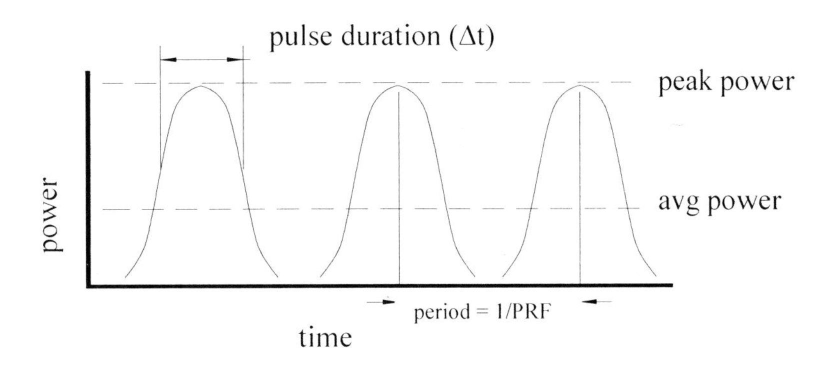

Figure D-1. Pulsed Laser Properties

D.11.5 Assigning a Laser Hazard Class. Determine the laser hazard class by comparing the effective power or energy per pulse (power or energy measured through a specific aperture) to the appropriate AEL for each class for each set of measurement conditions. The overall laser hazard class is the most restrictive of all applicable measurement conditions for all applicable time durations up to T_{max}.

D12. Hazard Evaluation.

Laser hazards are determined at locations where someone could be exposed to the laser radiation. Often, the exposure distance is not known for a particular laser. Therefore, it is usual practice to calculate a nominal ocular hazard distance (NOHD). For direct small-source viewing of the laser source, the MPE is exceeded at points within the beam at distances less than the NOHD, but not at greater distances. Note that it may be possible to not exceed the MPE at close ranges to the output of a focused beam. An NOHD may be computed both for unaided viewing and optically aided viewing. A nominal skin hazard distance (NSHD) is calculated for skin exposure. Exposure conditions for hazard evaluation may vary with distance, and must be updated for each evaluation distance considered.

D.12.1 Diffuse Reflection Hazards. Some high-power lasers can produce a hazard from diffuse reflections. The reflectivity of the target material is generally assumed to be 100% and the viewing angle is generally taken to be normal to the surface to simplify calculations. For close-in viewing of diffuse reflections (when the angular subtense of the diffuse image is greater than 1.5 mrad), the MPE can be calculated based on an extended source. When this applies, it is important to consider that the extended-source MPE decreases with distance since the angular subtense decreases.

D.12.2 Specular Reflection Hazards. The reflected beam properties from a material depend on the laser parameters and the characteristics of the material. Flat, specular reflectors in the laser beam path can greatly increase the NHZ of the laser (the locations where hazardous exposure could occur). Curved reflectors will alter the angular distribution of the beam and may increase the hazard near the reflector (for concave reflectors) but do not typically further increase the NHZ. Radiometric measurement may be required at the location of exposure to determine the actual level of hazard.

D.12.3 Skin Exposure. The MPE for the skin is provided in Table 7 of ANSI Z136.1-2007; however, for lengthy exposures exceeding 100 cm^2 of skin, the MPE may be reduced by as much as a factor of 10 (consult Section 8.4.2 of ANSI Z136.1-2007). In the retinal hazard region, the skin MPE is usually considerably higher (less restrictive) than the MPE for the eye. The limiting aperture diameter is 3.5 mm for skin, except for wavelengths longer than 100 μm (See Table 1 in this document). The value of t_{min} is often much less for skin hazards than ocular hazards; and therefore, determination of pulse width is more critical. Under some circumstances (e.g.,. for lasers operating between 1.5 and 1.8 μm), it is possible to exceed the skin MPE without exceeding the ocular MPE.

D.12.4 Irradiance and/or Radiant Exposure. The irradiance or radiant exposure averaged over the limiting apertures at all potential viewing distances is necessary for a complete hazard evaluation. When the viewing distance is far from the laser, where the laser beam diameter is much larger than the limiting aperture, the center beam irradiance or radiant exposure is adequate for assessing hazards.

D.12.5 Protective Eyewear. When the laser irradiance or radiant exposure exceeds the MPE, the required protection may be computed from the ratio of irradiance or radiant exposure and the MPE. The optical density, D_λ, (also called OD) may be computed from the $\log_{10}$ of the ratio of the irradiance or radiant exposure (averaged over the limiting aperture) and the MPE. Another method for computing the required OD is to compare the power or energy measured through the measurement aperture to the exposure limit in terms of power or energy based on the exposure duration used in the hazard evaluation Class 1 AEL (or 0.25-second exposure limit for visible laser beams), for either viewing condition and based on the intended viewing duration. When more than one wavelength is involved, protection at each wavelength must be assured and the additive effects of multiple wavelength exposure must also be taken into account.

Appendix E
Examples

E1. Detector Selection Example 1.

A pulsed Nd:YAG laser system has the manufacturer specified output parameters shown in Table E1-1. A measurement of laser pulse energy is required, but only three detectors are available for use. The detector specifications are listed in Table E1-2. Determine if any of the detectors can be used for a direct measurement of the laser pulse energy in two instances: (1) The laser beam expander is attached, (2) it is unattached.

Table E1-1. Laser Beam Parameters for Example 1

Parameter	Value (Case 1 with beam expander)	Value (Case 2 without beam expander)
Average Output Power	22 W	25 W
Exit Beam Profile	Gaussian	Gaussian
PRF	20 Hz	20 Hz
Pulse Duration	20 ns	20 ns
Exit Beam Dia. ($1/e^2$) irradiance pts.	3.0 cm	1.0 cm
Beam Divergence ($1/e^2$) irradiance pts.	0.5 mrad	1.5 mrad
Wavelength	1064 nm	1064 nm

Table E1-2. Detector Specifications for Example 1

Parameter	Detector 1	Detector 2	Detector 3
Max. Power (continuous)	30 W	150 W	30 W
Max. Intermittent Power	60 W	300 W	60 W
Min. Power Resolution	10 mW	10 mW	10 mW
Max. Average Irradiance	$26\ \text{kW}\cdot\text{cm}^{-2}$	$26\ \text{kW}\cdot\text{cm}^{-2}$	$26\ \text{kW}\cdot\text{cm}^{-2}$
Max. Pulse Radiant Exposure (20ns pulse)	$0.6\ \text{J}\cdot\text{cm}^{-2}$	$0.6\ \text{J}\cdot\text{cm}^{-2}$	$10\ \text{J}\cdot\text{cm}^{-2}$
Accuracy	+/- 3%	+/- 5%	+/- 3%
Clear Aperture	19 mm	50 mm	19 mm

To determine the appropriate detector, the parameters for comparison with the values listed in the detector specifications must first be determined. Then the comparison can be made to determine the appropriate detector for each case.

Case 1 with beam expander: Detector 2 is our most likely candidate because it is the only detector available with an input aperture of sufficient size. The maximum power handled by detector 2 is sufficient (150 W). To determine the power density (irradiance, E) and energy density (radiant exposure, H) values present, we divide the average power and pulse energies by the area of the beam. To obtain the peak value, we use the 1/e irradiance point beam diameter (a) in the Gaussian beam profile. To convert from the $1/e^2$ irradiance point commonly provided by manufacturers, we divide by $\sqrt{2}$.

$$a = \frac{3.0\ \text{cm}}{\sqrt{2}}$$

$$a = 2.1\ \text{cm}$$

and the peak average irradiance is

$$E_{\text{peak}} = \frac{4\ \Phi}{\pi\ a^2}$$

$$E_{\text{peak}} = \frac{4(22\text{W})}{\pi\ (2.1\ \text{cm})^2}$$

$$E_{\text{peak}} = 6.35\ \ \text{W/cm}^2$$

This is significantly lower than the $26\ \text{kW}\cdot\text{cm}^{-2}$ specification for all of the detectors. However, the value for the per-pulse energy must also be considered. The energy per pulse is simply the average output power divided by the number of pulses per second.

$$Q = \frac{\Phi}{\text{PRF}}$$

$$Q = \frac{22 \text{ W}}{20 \text{ Hz}}$$

$$Q = 1.1 \text{ J}$$

This divided by the beam area at the 1/e radiant exposure point gives us the peak radiant exposure (H_{peak}) on the detector face.

$$H_{\text{peak}} = \frac{4\ Q}{\pi\ a^2}$$

$$H_{\text{peak}} = \frac{4(1.1 \text{ J})}{\pi\ (2.1 \text{ cm})^2}$$

$$H_{\text{peak}} = 0.32\ \text{J/cm}^2$$

This is also less than the maximum pulse radiant exposure for the detectors which are rated at 0.6 $\text{J}\cdot\text{cm}^{-2}$ and 10 $\text{J}\cdot\text{cm}^{-2}$. The final consideration is the amount of clipping that occurs. If we assume that the beam profile is a perfect Gaussian, the fraction (δ) that is collected by the clear aperture of the detector can be determined from the following equation.

$$\delta = 1 - \exp\left(-\left(\frac{D_f}{D_L}\right)^2\right)$$

$$\delta = 1 - \exp\left(-\left(\frac{5.0 \text{ cm}}{2.1 \text{ cm}}\right)^2\right)$$

$$\delta = 0.997$$

So that 99.7% of the energy will be collected within the clear aperture of the detector. Therefore detector 2 is appropriate for the application. Note that applying the same equation to the two detectors with 19 mm apertures produces a value of 56% of the energy collected, making detectors 1 and 3 inappropriate for this measurement.

Case 2 without beam expander: Here it appears that all of the detectors available have an input aperture of sufficient size. The maximum power handled by all three detectors is sufficient (>25 W). Again, to determine the power density (irradiance, E) and energy density (radiant exposure H) values present, we divide the average power and pulse energies by the area of the beam. To obtain the peak value present, we again use the 1/e irradiance point beam diameter (a) in the Gaussian beam profile.

$$E_{\text{peak}} = \frac{4\ \Phi}{\pi\ a^2}$$

$$E_{\text{peak}} = \frac{4(25\ \text{W})}{\pi\ (0.71\ \text{cm})^2}$$

$$E_{\text{peak}} = 63\ \ \text{W/cm}^2$$

This is significantly lower than the 26 $\text{kW}\cdot\text{cm}^{-2}$ specification. However, the value for the per pulse energy must also be considered. The energy per pulse is simply the average output power divided by the number of pulses per second.

$$Q = \frac{\Phi}{\text{PRF}}$$

$$Q = \frac{25\ \text{W}}{20\ \text{Hz}}$$

$$Q = 1.25\ \text{J}$$

This divided by the beam area at the 1/e radiant exposure point gives us the peak radiant exposure (H_{peak}) on the detector face.

$$H_{\text{peak}} = \frac{4\ Q}{\pi\ a^2}$$

$$H_{\text{peak}} = \frac{4(1.25\ \text{J})}{\pi\ (0.71\ \text{cm})^2}$$

$$H_{\text{peak}} = 3.2\ \ \text{J/cm}^2$$

This peak radiant exposure value eliminates all detectors except detector 3. Detector 3 has a maximum pulse radiant exposure of 10 $\text{J}\cdot\text{cm}^{-2}$, sufficient for this application.

The final consideration is the amount of clipping that occurs for detector 3, which has a clear aperture of 19 mm. If we assume that the beam profile is a perfect Gaussian, the fraction (δ) of energy from the beam that is collected by the clear aperture of the detector is calculated from the following equation.

$$\delta = 1 - \exp\left(-\left(\frac{D_f}{D_L} \right)^2 \right)$$

$$\delta = 1 - \exp\left(-\left(\frac{1.9\ \text{cm}}{0.71\ \text{cm}} \right)^2 \right)$$

$$\delta = 0.999$$

Since 99.9% of the energy will be collected within the clear aperture of the detector, detector 3 is appropriate for the application.

E2. Detector Selection Example 2.

A high repetition-rate laser system has the manufacturer specified output parameters shown in Table E2-1. A measurement of laser pulse power is required to confirm the divergence using the knife-edge technique, but only three detectors are available for use. The detector manufacturer's specifications are listed in Table E2-2. Determine if any of the detectors can be used for a direct measurement of the laser output power.

Table E2-1. Laser Beam Parameters for Example 2

Parameter	Specified Value
Wavelength	1.55 µm
Average Pulse Energy	30 µJ
Exit Beam Profile	Gaussian
PRF	1.0 kHz
Pulse Duration	500 ns
Exit Beam Dia. ($1/e^2$) radiant exposure pts.	0.53 cm
Beam Divergence ($1/e^2$) radiant exposure pts.	0.4 mrad

Table E2-2. Detector Specifications for Example 2

Parameter	Detector 1	Detector 2	Detector 3
Detector Type	Silicon (Si)	Germanium (Ge)	Pyroelectric
Max. Power (continuous)	1 W	10 mW	2 W
Min. Power Resolution	0.5 μW	10 nW	1 mW
Max. Average Power Density	0.5 W·cm^{-2}	0.5 W·cm^{-2}	26 kW·cm^{-2}
Max Radiant Exposure	--	--	< 100 ns 0.1 J cm^{-2} 1 μs 0.2 J cm^{-2} 300 μs 4 J cm^{-2}
Max Pulse Energy	50 μJ	5 μJ	--
Max PRF	CW	CW	4000 Hz
Accuracy	+/- 5%	+/- 5%	+/- 3%
Clear Aperture	8 mm	5 mm	19 mm

To determine the appropriate detector, the parameters for comparison with the values listed in the detector specifications must first be determined. Then the comparison can be made to determine the appropriate detector for each case. Notice the repetition rate is 1 kHz, which is within the specifications of all three detectors. A measure of average power can be used to compute the energy per pulse. Using an oscilloscope, the pulse repetition frequency can be measured with a different instrument than used to measure total output power or energy. Next, notice that the wavelength is 1.55 μm, which will be a factor in detector selection.

First do a quick calculation of the expected power output. The manufacturer specified a pulse energy of 30 μJ per pulse and a 1 kHz pulse repetition frequency. To get average power, we multiply the pulse energy by PRF.

The estimated average power from the laser is $\Phi = Q \cdot \text{PRF} = (30 \times 10^{-6}\ \text{J})(1 \times 10^{3}\ \text{Hz}) = 30\ \text{mW}$.

Now, consider the wavelength of the laser. By looking at the wavelength response curves for the silicon, germanium and pyroelectric detectors listed in the detectors manuals (see also Figure 1 in the main body of this document), we immediately eliminate the silicon detector from consideration because its nominal wavelength response range is 400 nm-1100 nm. By checking the wavelength response of the germanium (800 nm to 1800 nm) and pyroelectric (200 nm to 5 μm) detectors, we determine that both of these detectors have sensitivity at 1.55 μm.

Next, by comparing the expected output of 30 mW to the maximum power, we determine that the germanium detector (detector 2) will not handle the power output or the energy output of the laser; however, it can be used to measure the PRF by collecting only a small portion of the output power. Next, we compare the maximum irradiance allowed on detector 3.

To determine the irradiance, we divide the average power by the area of the beam. To obtain the peak value present, we use the 1/e irradiance point beam diameter (a) in the Gaussian beam profile. To convert from the 1/e^2 irradiance point commonly provided by manufacturers, we divide by √2.

$$a = \frac{0.53 \text{ cm}}{\sqrt{2}}$$

$$a = 0.375 \text{ cm}$$

and the peak average irradiance is:

$$E_{\text{peak}} = \frac{4\Phi}{\pi a^2}$$

$$E_{\text{peak}} = \frac{4(30 \times 10^{-3} \text{ W})}{\pi (0.375 \text{ cm})^2}$$

$$E_{\text{peak}} = 0.271 \text{ W/cm}^2$$

This is significantly lower than the 26 kW·cm^{-2} maximum average power specification for detector 3. However, the value for the per-pulse energy must also be considered. The energy divided by the beam area at the 1/e intensity point gives us the peak radiant exposure (H_{peak}) on the detector face.

$$H_{\text{peak}} = \frac{4Q}{\pi a^2}$$

$$H_{\text{peak}} = \frac{4(30 \times 10^{-6} \text{ J})}{\pi (0.375 \text{ cm})^2}$$

$$H_{\text{peak}} = 0.27 \text{ mJ/cm}^2$$

This peak radiant exposure value does not exceed the maximum for pulses on the order of 1 µs in duration, which is 200 mJ·cm^{-2}, sufficient for this application.

The final consideration is the amount of clipping that occurs. If we assume that the beam profile is a perfect Gaussian, the fraction (δ) that is collected by the clear aperture of the detector can be determined from the following equation.

$$\delta = 1 - e^{\left(-\left(\frac{D_f}{D_L}\right)^2\right)}$$

$$\delta = 1 - e^{\left(-\left(\frac{1.9}{0.375}\right)^2\right)}$$

$\delta = 1$

The clear aperture of the detector will collect 100% of the energy. Therefore, detector 3 is appropriate for the application.

E3. Selecting Measurement Apertures.

Table E3-1 lists five laboratory lasers, built "in-house," to be used for experiments indoors and outdoors. Determine the measurement apertures needed for classification of each laser.

Table E3-1. Laser Parameters for Example 3

Parameter	Laser 1	Laser 2	Laser 3	Laser 4	Laser 5
Wavelength	0.532 μm	0.633 μm	1.064 μm	10.600 μm	49.600 μm
Diameter	2 cm	0.3 cm	1 cm	10 cm	10 cm
Divergence	6 mrad	10 mrad	0.5 mrad	1 mrad	1 mrad
Pulsed or CW	CW	CW	Pulsed	CW	CW
PRF	N/A	N/A	30 Hz	N/A	N/A
Pulse Duration	N/A	N/A	20 ns	N/A	N/A

In order to choose a measurement aperture, we need to know the wavelength, the exposure duration and whether optical aids could be used with the laser.

Laser 1: Since this laser is in the visible spectrum, we must determine whether optical aids will present a more severe optical hazard than unaided viewing. Condition 2, from Table 9 in ANSI Z136.1-2007, lists an aperture diameter of 7.0 mm and a measurement distance of 10 cm for all exposure durations. Since the beam diameter is 2 cm, optical aids must be taken into account. Condition 1, from Table 9 in ANSI Z136.1-2007, lists an aperture diameter of 50.0 mm and a measurement distance of 200 cm.

Laser 2: Again, since this laser is in the visible spectrum, we must determine whether optical aids will present a more severe optical hazard than unaided viewing. Condition 2, from Table 9 in ANSI Z136.1-2007, lists an aperture diameter of 7.0 mm and a measurement distance of 10 cm for all exposure durations. Since the beam diameter is 0.3 cm, optical aids need not be taken into account, because all the power in the beam enters the eye without optical aids near the exit port. Therefore, optical aids would just attenuate the beam relative to unaided viewing. Thus, the measurement aperture for classification of this laser is 7.0 mm. However, optical aids will extend the NOHD.

Laser 3: This laser is in the near-infrared part of the spectrum, but for determining the measurement aperture, we have the same case as the visible part of the spectrum because this wavelength is still focused by optics and the eye. Condition 2, from Table 9 in ANSI Z136.1-2007, lists an aperture diameter of 7.0 mm and a measurement distance of 10 cm for all exposure durations. Since the beam diameter is 1 cm, optical aids must be taken into account. Condition 1, from Table 9 in ANSI Z136.1-2007, lists an aperture diameter of 50.0 mm and a measurement distance of 200 cm.

Laser 4: This laser is in the far-infrared part of the spectrum. A note in Table 9 of ANSI Z136.1-2007 states that Condition 1 does not apply for lasers having wavelengths exceeding 2.8 μm since most telescopic optics do not transmit beyond 2.8 μm. Therefore, we do not need to be concerned with optical aids. However, exposure duration is needed to determine the measurement aperture. For the sake of safety, let's assume a 10 s exposure duration as ANSI Z136.1-2007 provides. Condition 2, from Table 9 of ANSI Z136.1-2007, lists an aperture diameter of either 1.0, $1.5t^{0.375}$, or 3.5 mm. However, there is a note in the table that says that under normal conditions, the exposure duration from 0.3 to 10 s would not be used for classification, so the aperture diameter for this laser is 3.5 mm since the laser is CW. For repetitively pulsed lasers, either a 1.0 mm or 3.5 mm measurement aperture may be appropriate, depending on whether the hazard originates from individual pulses or average power.

Laser 5: This laser is in the far-infrared part of the spectrum. A note in Table 2 (Table 9 of ANSI Z136.1-2007) states that Condition 1 does not apply for lasers having wavelengths exceeding 2.8 μm since most telescopic optics do not transmit beyond 2.8 μm. Therefore, we do not need to be concerned with optical aids. Condition 2, from Table 9 of ANSI Z136.1-2007, lists an aperture diameter of 11.0 and a measurement distance of 10 cm for all exposure durations, so the measurement aperture for this laser is 11.0 mm.

E4. Energy Measurement.

Noise-Equivalent Energy: A pulsed Nd:YAG laser system is anticipated to have a low energy per pulse output. Describe the lowest pulse energy that can be reliably measured with a pyroelectric joulemeter probe and radiometer combination with a voltage response (R_v) of 2.5 V/mJ and a noise equivalent voltage (NEV) of 3.75 μV.

The ratio of the above parameters can be used to compute a noise equivalent joule (NEJ) of pulse energy. In this case:

$$\text{NEJ} = \frac{\text{NEV}}{R_v}$$

$$\text{NEJ} = \frac{3.75 \times 10^{-6}\ \text{V}}{2.5 \times 10^{-3}\ \dfrac{\text{V}}{\text{J}}}$$

$$\text{NEJ} = 1.5 \times 10^{-9}\ \text{J} = 1.5\ \text{nJ}$$

E5. Classification.

Using the guidelines found in Section 4.2 determine the classification of the three lasers with parameters listed in Table E5-1.

Table E5-1. Laser Output Parameters for Example 5

Parameter	Laser 1	Laser 2	Laser 3
Average Output Power	525 mW	150 mW	30 mW
Output Energy per Pulse	N/A	N/A	30 nJ
Beam Divergence ($1/e^2$) irradiance points	0.5 mrad	0.8 mrad	0.4 mrad
Exit Beam Diameter ($1/e^2$) irradiance points	2.6 cm	1.0 mm	1.0 cm
Exit Beam Profile	Gaussian	Gaussian	Gaussian
Output Type	CW	CW	Pulsed
PRF	N/A	N/A	1.0 MHz
Pulse Duration	N/A	N/A	500 ns
Wavelength	870 nm	532 nm	1550 nm
Beam Waist Location	20 m	Output Aperture	Output Aperture
Diameter Beam Waist ($1/e^2$) irradiance points	1.9 cm	N/A	N/A
Source Size	$<\alpha_{min}$	$<\alpha_{min}$	N/A
Intended Use	IR Illuminator for US Military Outdoor Use	High Power Visible Pointer for Outdoor Use	Indoor Motion Detection System

Laser 1: Determine limits for each class

Unaided Viewing

a.) Class 1 and Class 1M

The time base used for a Class 1 system is 100 s. ANSI Z136.1-2007 indicates that the AEL for emission in the wavelength range 700 nm -1050 nm with an exposure duration in the range from 10 s to 3×10^4 s and with $\alpha \leq \alpha_{min}$ is given by:

$$AEL_{Class1} = 3.9 \times 10^{-4} C_A \text{ W}$$

From Table 6 (ANSI), $C_A = 10^{2(\lambda-0.700)} = 2.19$ and hence $AEL_{Class1} = 8.5 \times 10^{-4}$ W. This must be compared with the power collected through the measurement aperture. The appropriate limiting aperture for this laser is 7.0 mm for the eye and 3.5 mm for the skin. The $1/e^2$ beam diameter at the output of the laser is given as 2.6 cm. Since there is a beam waist, the size at the beam waist is used since this is the most hazardous position. This yields a 1/e beam diameter of 1.3 cm.

The fraction of the total emitted power that passes through the measurement aperture for unaided viewing is

$$\Phi_a = \left[1 - e^{-\left(\frac{0.7}{1.3}\right)^2}\right]\Phi_o = 132 \text{ mW}$$

The laser output exceeds the Class 1 limit. Since the Class 1 limit is exceeded, the Class 1M limit does not need to be checked.

b.) Class 2 and Class 2M

Class 2 and Class 2M apply only to visible lasers.

c.) Class 3R

The Class 3R limit is 5 times the Class 1 limit. For this example, that would be

$$AEL_{Class3R} = 5 \cdot (\Phi_{Class1}) = 4.25 \text{ mW}$$

The laser output exceeds the Class 3R limit.

d.) Class 3B

The 132 mW measured is compared with the Class 3B AEL of 500 mW for exposures exceeding 0.25 s. Because the 132 mW does not exceed this value, Laser 1 is an ANSI Class 3B laser system based on unaided viewing.

Aided Viewing

The appropriate measurement aperture for this laser is 50.0 mm as the laser is intended for outdoor military use where binocular viewing is possible. The beam waist is located at 20 m, so a 20-m measurement distance is used. A measurement of maximum output power through a measurement aperture of 50.0 mm during T_{max} with losses due to transmission through the optics considered yields 367 mW, as shown

$$\Phi_a = 0.7\left[1 - e^{-\left(\frac{5.0}{1.3}\right)^2}\right]\Phi_o = 367 \text{ mW}$$

Summary

The hazard class is Class 3B based on the worst case of unaided and optically aided viewing.

Laser 2: Determine limits for each class

Unaided Viewing

a.) Class 1 and Class 1M

The time base used for a Class 1 system is 30,000 s. It can be shown that the AEL for emission in the wavelength range 400 nm to 700 nm with an exposure duration in the range from 10 s to 3×10^4 s and with $\alpha \leq \alpha_{min}$ is given by:

$$\text{AEL}_{\text{Class1}} = 3.9 \times 10^{-4} \text{ W}$$

This must be compared with the power collected through the measurement aperture. The appropriate limiting aperture for this laser is 7.0 mm for the eye and 3.5 mm for the skin. The $1/e^2$ beam diameter at the output of the laser is given as 1.0 mm. This yields a 1/e beam diameter of 0.7 mm. Since the diameter of the beam at the output is so much smaller than the limiting aperture, all the power passes through the limiting aperture.

$$\Phi_a = \left[1 - e^{-\left(\frac{0.7}{0.07}\right)^2}\right]\Phi_o = 150 \text{ mW}$$

The laser output exceeds the Class 1 limit, and the Class 1M limit does not need to be checked.

b.) Class 2 and Class 2M

The time base used for a Class 2 system is 0.25 s. ANSI Z136.1-2007 indicates that the AEL for emission in the wavelength range 400 nm to 700 nm with an exposure duration in the range from 1×10^{-3} to 0.35 s is

$$\text{AEL}_{\text{Class2}} = 1.0 \text{ mW}$$

The laser output exceeds the Class 2 limit, so the Class 2M limit does not need to be checked.

c.) Class 3R

The Class 3R limits are 5 times the Class 2 limits. For this example, that would be

$$AEL_{class3R} = 5 \cdot (AEL_{Class2}) = 5 \text{ mW}$$

The laser output exceeds the Class 3R limit.

d.) Class 3B

The 150 mW measured is compared with the Class 3B AEL of 500 mW for exposures exceeding 0.25 s. Because the 150 mW does not exceed this value, Laser 2 is an ANSI Class 3B laser system based on unaided viewing.

Aided Viewing

The appropriate measurement aperture for this laser is 50.0 mm as the laser is intended for outdoor use where binocular viewing is possible. A measurement of maximum output power through a measurement aperture of 50.0 mm during T_{max} with losses due to transmission through the optics considered yields 135 mW, as shown

$$\Phi_a = 0.9\left[1 - e^{-\left(\frac{5.0}{0.07}\right)^2}\right]\Phi_o = 135 \text{ mW}$$

Summary

The hazard class is Class 3B based on the worst case of unaided and optically aided viewing.

Laser 3: Determine limits for each class

Unaided Viewing

a.) Class 1 and Class 1M

The time base used for a Class 1 system is 100 s. ANSI Z136.1-2007 indicates that the AEL for emission in the wavelength range 1400 nm to 4000 nm with an exposure duration in the range from 10 s to 3×10^4 s is given by:

$$AEL_{Class1} = 9.6 \times 10^{-3} \text{ W}$$

This must be compared with the power collected through the limiting aperture. The output can be treated like a CW emission at a power level equal to the average emitted power due to the high data transmission rate. The appropriate limiting aperture for this laser is 3.5 mm for both the eye and the skin. The $1/e^2$ beam diameter at the output of the laser is given as 1.0 cm. This yields a 1/e beam diameter of 0.7 cm.

$$\Phi_a = \left[1 - e^{-\left(\frac{0.35}{0.7}\right)^2}\right]\Phi_o = 6.6 \text{ mW}$$

The laser output does not exceed the Class 1 limit for unaided viewing.

Aided Viewing

The appropriate measurement aperture for this laser is 25.0 mm as the laser is intended for outdoor use where binocular viewing is possible. A measurement of maximum output power through a measurement aperture of 25.0 mm during T_{max} with losses due to transmission through the optics considered yields 21 mW, as shown

$$\Phi_a = 0.7\left[1 - e^{-\left(\frac{2.5}{0.7}\right)^2}\right]\Phi_o = 21\text{ mW}$$

This exceeds the Class 1 limit for aided viewing. 21 mW is compared with the Class 3B AEL of 500 mW. Because the 21 mW does not exceed this value, Laser 3 is an ANSI Class 1M laser system. However, the intended use of the system is for indoor motion detection, so we can generally assume that it will not be viewed with binoculars.

Summary

The hazard class is Class 1M based on the worst case of unaided and aided viewing.

E6. Beam Diameter, Beam Profile, Irradiance Distribution.

Examples E6a. and E6b. illustrate beam profiles in the near field that are Gaussian and non-Gaussian, respectively.

E6a. Gaussian Beam Profiles (Near Field)

The beam profiles shown in Figure E6-1 exhibit a circular beam profile in the case of Profile 1, or a small slit-shaped profile in the case of Profile 2. ISO 11146 Part 1 "4-Sigma" and Gaussian fit analyses were used as well as a Peak/Total Energy Gaussian and cylindrical models as shown in Figures E6-2 and E6-3. An analysis was also conducted by determining the size of circular aperture required to transmit 90% or 70% of the total energy for Profiles 1 and 2, respectively.

The resulting analyses, as listed in Table E6-1, indicate that ISO 11146 Part 1 and Gaussian Fit Measurement methods of beam characterization are fairly accurate models of the peak exposure levels ($J\cdot cm^{-2}$) at the output aperture of the lasers. In the ISO 11146 Part 1 and Gaussian Fit techniques, the measured energy emitted per square centimeter disagree with modeled values by about 10-30%. However, because the Peak/Total Energy method is constrained to match the peak energy level, the prediction of maximum exposure is most accurate in terms of laser exposure level, and is in good agreement with the other two techniques (10-20% for both lasers). It is important to observe that in the near-field profiles, the peak exposure criteria for determining equivalent diameter is not peak pixel in the respective profiles, but is the exposure transmitted through a 7-mm circular aperture. This is a criterion for hazard analysis, used in the ANSI Z136.1-2007 Standard. Consequently, peaks in the models will not correspond to the peak in the profile if the beam is very small (<0.7 cm in diameter).

Table E6-1. Beam Profile Analysis Results

Measurement Method	Profile 1 Beam Diameter (cm)	Profile 2 Beam Diameter (cm)
ISO 11146 – 4 Sigma ($1/e^2$)	3.43 ± 0.08	0.96 ± 0.07
Gaussian Fit ($1/e^2$)	4.01 ± 0.14	1.14 ± 0.07
Peak/Total Energy Equivalent Gaussian ($1/e^2$)	4.35 ± 0.16	1.24 ± 0.09
90%/70% Transmission Aperture	3.33 ± 0.08	0.62 ± 0.08

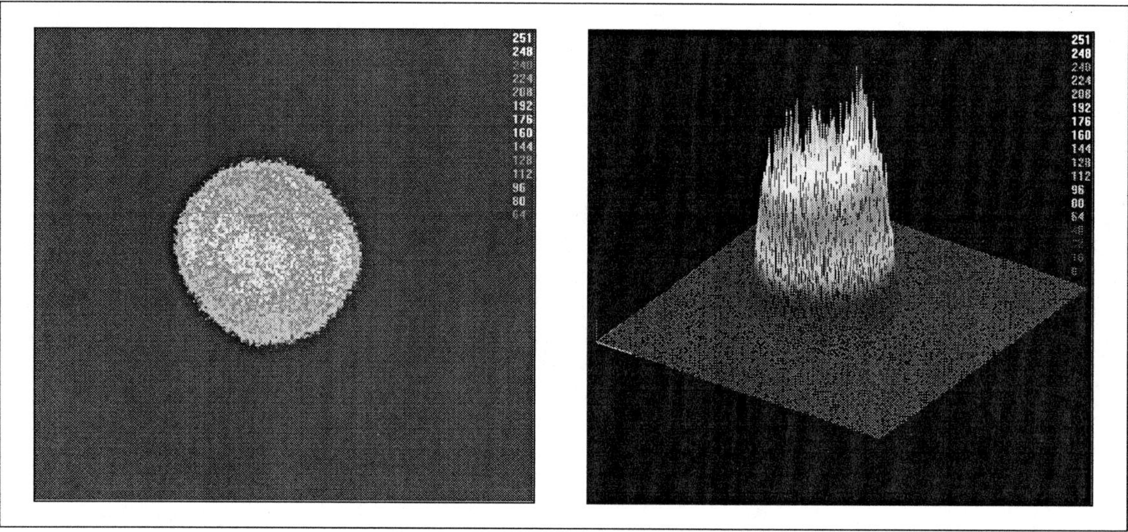

Profile 1. Near Field Profile

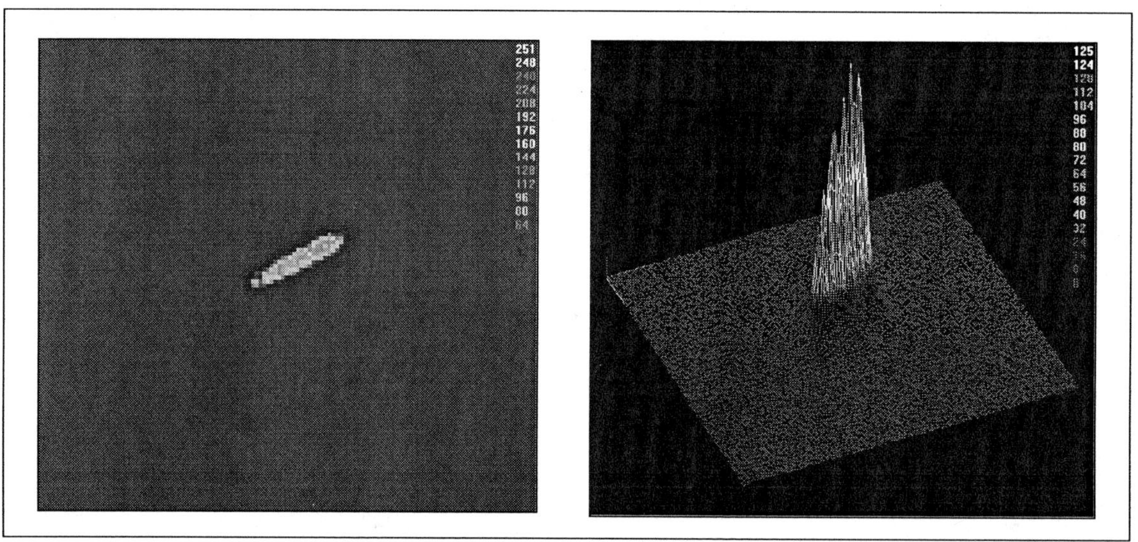

Profile 2. Near Field Profile

Figure E6-1. Near Field Beam Profiles 1 and 2

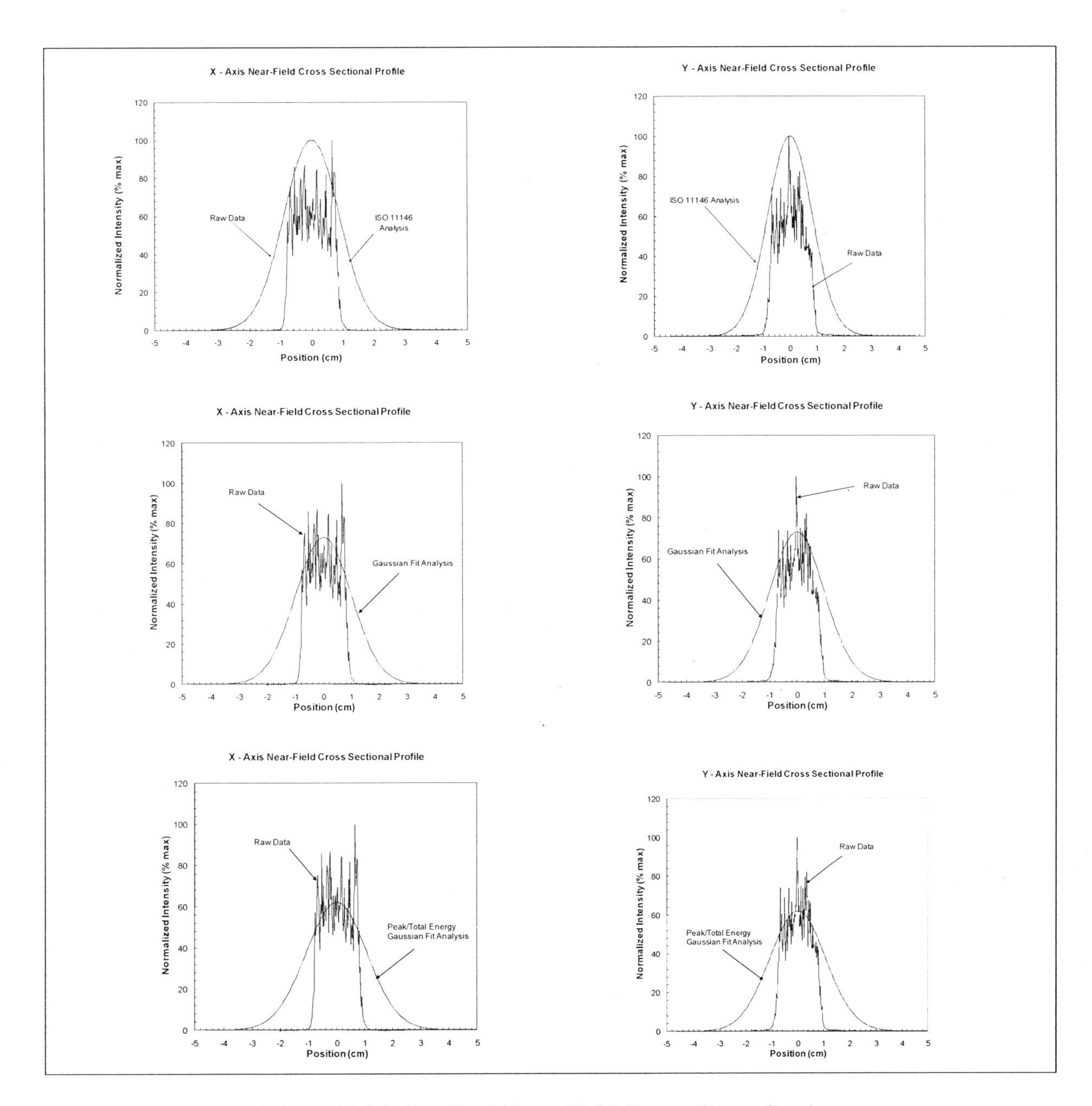

Figure E6-2. Profile 1 Near Field Beam Cross-Section

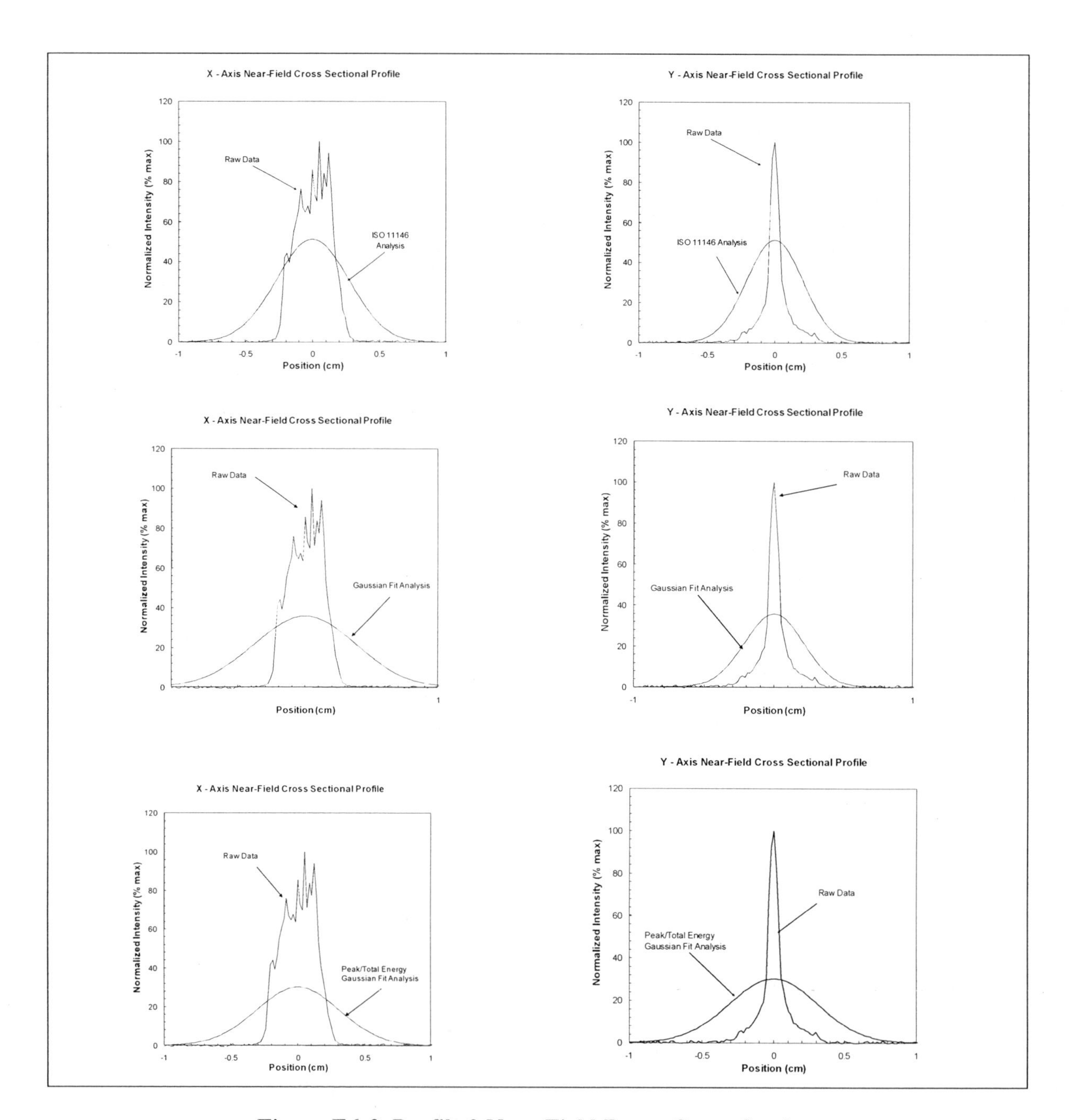

Figure E6-3. Profile 2 Near Field Beam Cross-Section

E6b. Non-Gaussian Beam Profiles (Near Field)

Many lasers do not have a beam profile that is well approximated by a Gaussian distribution. In these cases, it is necessary to find alternate methods of characterization that accurately determine hazard parameters.

> *NOTE: The near field region is the area closest to an aperture or source where the diffraction pattern differs substantially from that observed at an infinite distance. This is the region of Fresnel diffraction.*

Consider a Q-Switched Nd:YAG laser (1.064 µm) that has the cross-sectional beam profiles illustrated in Figure E6-4. The beam profile is measured one meter from the output aperture and the cross sections are taken through the peak of the profile. The total energy in each pulse is 100 millijoules. Describe methods that can be used to accurately determine or specify laser exposure.

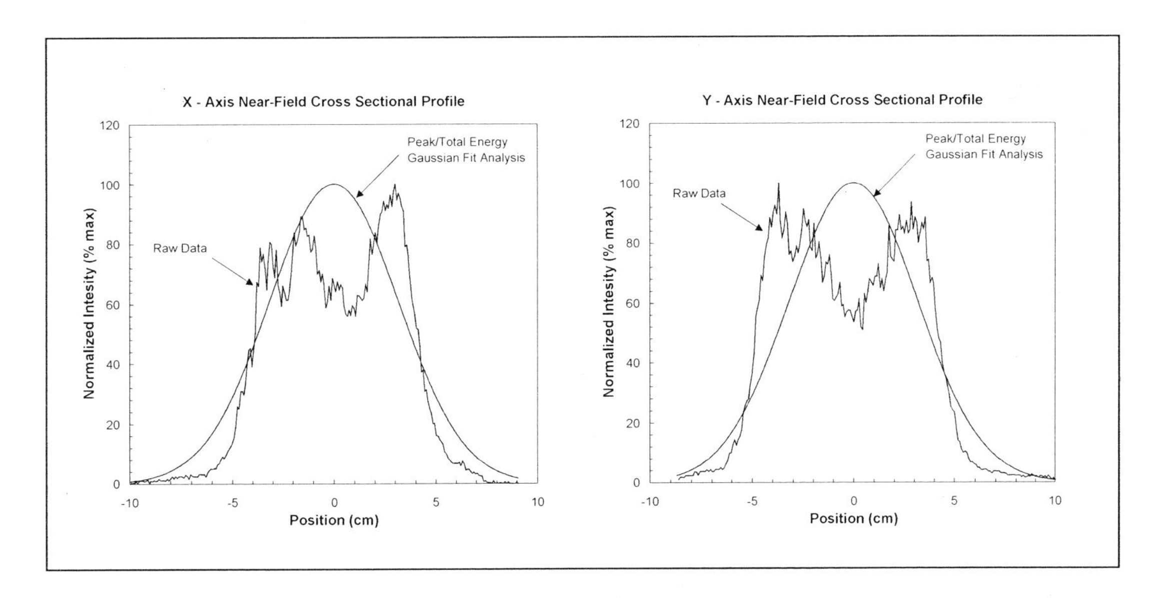

Figure E6-4. Beam Cross-Section for Example 6

Table E6-2. Data for Example 6

Method	0.7 cm Aperture Exposure	Radiant Exposure	"1/e" Beam Diameter
Energy Transmitted - Fixed Aperture	590 µJ	1.5 mJ·cm^{-2}	9.2 cm
Beam Profiler – Software Analysis	605 µJ	1.7 mJ·cm^{-2}	9.0 cm
Gaussian Fit – Least Squares Method	920 µJ	2.2 mJ·cm^{-2}	7.6 cm
ISO 11146 – Standard Computation	970 µJ	2.5 mJ·cm^{-2}	7.1 cm

(1) ***Aperture Methods.*** In the absence of electronic beam-profiling equipment, exposures can be well characterized by measuring laser energy transmitted through a fixed aperture. If we are interested in the unaided viewing hazards from this laser, a 0.7 cm fixed aperture can be used to measure exposure, and compute an "equivalent" beam diameter that can be used for other computations. The aperture must be scanned in both directions across the beam to obtain the highest reading, which indicates maximum hazard.

In this example, a measurement of total pulse energy yields 100 mJ. The energy measured through a 0.7 cm diameter fixed aperture yields 590 μJ from which an average exposure over the aperture's area yields 1.5 mJ·cm^{-2}.

Comparison of the beam size to the 0.7 cm aperture shows that the aperture is sampling only a very small portion of the beam. This means that the exposure should be fairly constant over the aperture area. A Gaussian Beam profile with equivalent total energy per pulse and a corresponding peak radiant energy of 1.5 mJ·cm^{-2} would have a "1/e" diameter determined from the equation:

$$D_L = \sqrt{\frac{4Q}{\pi H}}$$

$$D_L = \sqrt{\frac{4 \cdot (100 \text{ mJ})}{\pi \cdot (1.5 mJ \cdot cm^{-2})}}$$

$$D_L = 9.2 \text{ cm}$$

(2) ***Beam Profile Software Analyses.*** Several analysis techniques may be applied to data captured from a laser profiler. Here we will examine the results from (a) software generation of an "artificial aperture," (b) a "least-squares" Gaussian functional fit to the cross-section data, and (c) an ISO 11146 analysis.

(a) The software used to capture the profiles can compute the peak exposure and can also compute the energy transmitted through an area of a fixed aperture. In this example, the software yields 1.7 mJ·cm^{-2} for the peak pixel irradiance value and 605 μJ for the energy transmitted through the fixed aperture simulated by the software. The value of 1.7 mJ·cm^{-2} is compared with the average radiant exposure over the 0.7 cm aperture computed from the equation:

$$H = \frac{4\,Q}{\pi\,a^2}$$

The radiant exposure is computed to be 1.6 mJ·cm^{-2}, in good agreement with the 1.7 mJ·cm^{-2} computed from the peak pixel value. This indicates that the assumption from the fixed aperture measurement is valid and that the irradiance is fairly constant over the aperture.

(b) The beam profiler software package also has the option of computing a "least-squares" Gaussian functional fit to the data. This functional fit provides an approximation to the beam and can be used to compute a peak exposure from the fit parameters.

The Gaussian fit yields an average beam diameter of 7.6 cm at the "1/e" irradiance point. The fit also determines a peak irradiance value of 2.2 mJ·cm^{-2}. Assuming that the beam has a Gaussian profile with these parameters yields a transmittance through a 0.7-cm aperture of:

$$Q_f = Q\left[1 - e^{\left(-\left(\frac{D_f}{D_L}\right)^2\right)}\right]$$

$$Q_f = 100\ \text{mJ}\left[1 - e^{\left(-\left(\frac{0.7\ \text{cm}}{7.6\ \text{cm}}\right)^2\right)}\right]$$

$$Q_f = 100\ \text{mJ}(0.0092)$$

$$Q_f = 920\ \mu\text{J}$$

This value is significantly larger than the measured value of 590 μJ, indicating that this method will *overestimate* exposure for this beam profile.

(c) The final method of determining beam parameters is the ISO 11146 analysis methodology. This method is well documented in the standard and can be used to determine beam parameters for any shape of beam profile, in a consistent, well-defined manner. However, the ISO standard was not designed for laser hazard analysis.

The application of the ISO 11146 characterization yields a "4-σ" beam diameter of 10 cm, which for a Gaussian distribution is a 7.1 cm beam diameter at the 1/e radiant exposure points. Assuming a Gaussian profile of this diameter and applying the equation above, one obtains an exposure of 970 μJ through a 0.7 cm fixed aperture. This value again is significantly larger than the 590 μJ measured directly.

Summary

The application of the methods above shows that the most accurate exposure computation is determined from either direct measurement or through computation of maximum exposure through software tools. In this case, the ISO 11146 and Gaussian functional fit methodologies obtained larger exposures than were actually present. This makes for a conservative hazard analysis in this particular instance, but could affect classification in some tests.

E7. Diode Laser Illuminator.

Non-Gaussian Beam Profiles (Far Field). Many lasers do not have a beam profile that is well approximated by a Gaussian distribution in the far-field. In these cases, it is necessary to find alternate methods of characterization that accurately determine hazard parameters. An inaccurate divergence value can have significant impact on NOHDs.

NOTE: The far field region is the area far from an aperture or source where the diffraction pattern is essentially the same as that at infinity. This is the region of Fraunhofer diffraction.

Here, we will consider two cases (a) a square beam projected in the far field from a diode laser illuminator and (b) an irregular beam profile that is not well described by any functional form. Comparisons will be made applying the methods described in the near field example.

(1) Consider a diode laser illuminator with the far-field profile as shown in Figure E7-1. The laser projects a profile that can be accurately represented as a "flat-top" profile that is square. This profile is measured by a laser beam profiler, capturing an image of the laser profile at the back focal plane of a large aperture, 1.9 m focal length lens. The image must be examined at the specified (or measured) geometric (or infinity) point of the lens and not the location of the smallest image. It is also important to verify the portion of the actual laser beam that is captured by the profiler. If the profile camera only collects a portion of the total emitted energy, inaccurate estimates of the downrange irradiance will be produced.

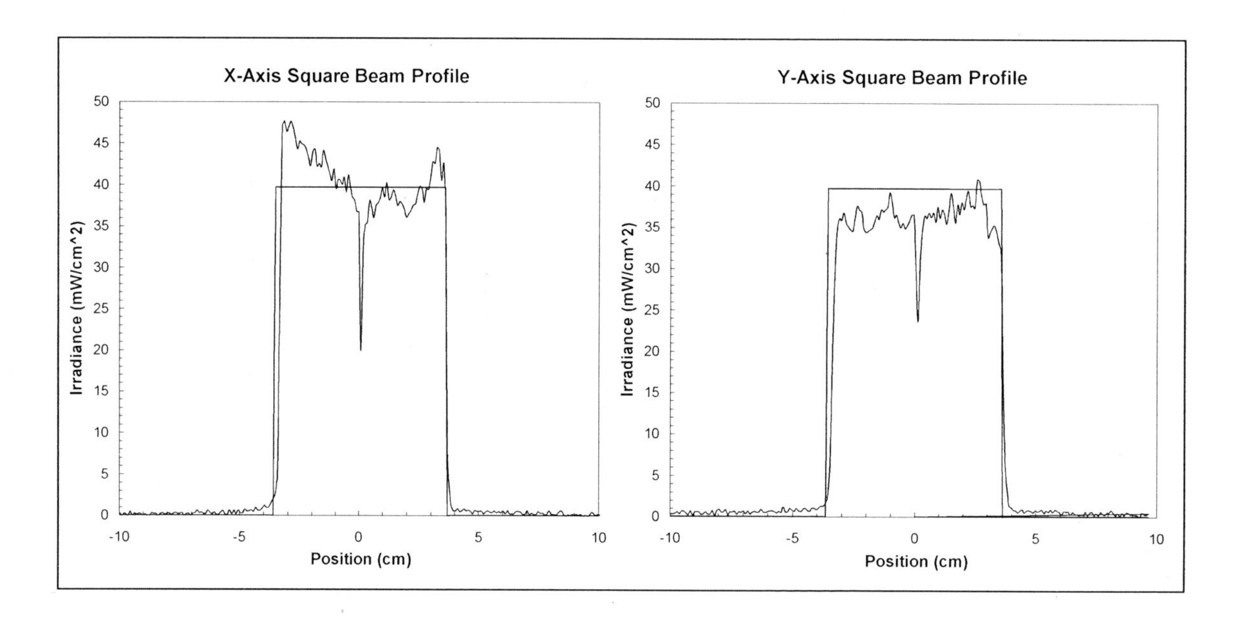

Figure E7-1. Far Field Profile – Diode Laser Illuminator

Because this laser can be modeled well with a "top-hat" or "flat-top" cross-sectional beam profile, the full width at half maximum is measured for the beam along the axes of the beam. It is determined that the beam size at the back focal plane of the lens is 7.1 cm × 7.1 cm. This yields a divergence of 3.7 mrad × 3.7 mrad from the equation:

$$\phi = \frac{d_f}{f},$$

where d_f is the diameter of the beam along either axis and f is the focal length of the lens. The total power in the beam is 2 W, so a functional profile can be drawn and compared with the raw data. Figure E7-1 shows this comparison near the centroid of the beam. The average irradiance within the square beam model is:

$$E = \frac{\Phi}{d_1 d_2},$$

where Φ is the total power of the beam (2 W), and d_1 and d_2 are the respective beam diameters of the two dimensions of the beam, in this case 7.1 cm. This average irradiance is approximately 40 mW·cm^{-2} and compares well with the peak irradiance within the spot profile of about 48 mW·cm^{-2}. This value, however, underestimates the peak exposure that an individual may receive by as much as 20%, the borderline of acceptable hazard analysis measurements, according to the ANSI Z136.1.

An alternate method that can be used to accurately determine far-field maximum irradiance, while sacrificing accuracy in far-field beam width is similar to the second method in example E6b, that is, to determine the *peak* pixel value and then compute an equivalent beam size. For the square beam containing 2 W of power and a peak pixel irradiance of 48 mW·cm^{-2}, the equation above used, solving for d_1 (assuming d_1 and d_2 are equal for the square beam) and one obtains 6.5 cm for an "equivalent" peak exposure beam diameter. This also yields a divergence value of 3.4 mrad for the beam, a difference of only about 0.6 cm in diameter (less than 10%), but producing a more precise exposure value in the far field. It should be noted that a 10% difference in diameter or divergence will produce over a 20% difference in corneal irradiance predictions.

An ISO 11146 analysis applied to this beam profile through profiler software methods, yields a beam diameter of 9.7 cm, a divergence of 5.1 mrad, and a peak irradiance of 47 mW·cm^{-2}. This irradiance value assumes a Gaussian distribution fit to the data. The ISO standard does accurately predict peak irradiance although a different far field distribution is being assumed. Data is provided in Table E7-1.

Table E7-1. Data for Example 7

Method	Profile Max Irradiance	Beam Diameter	Divergence
Beam Profiler – Peak Pixel Software Analysis	48 mW·cm^{-2}	6.5 cm	3.4 mrad
Square Fit – Least Squares Method	40 mW·cm^{-2}	7.1 cm	3.7 mrad
ISO 11146 – Standard Computation	47 mW·cm^{-2}	9.7 cm	5.1 mrad

In this example care must be taken when predicting far-field exposures and determining NOHD. In the instance of a square-beam (or rectangular-beam) profile, the equation describing exposure differs from that for a Gaussian profile by $\pi/4$:

$$H_{\text{gaussian}}(r) = \frac{4\Phi}{\pi\sqrt{\left(d_1^2 + \phi_1^2 r^2\right)\left(d_2^2 + \phi_2^2 r^2\right)}}$$

$$H_{\text{square}}(r) = \frac{\Phi}{\sqrt{\left(d_1^2 + \phi_1^2 r^2\right)\left(d_2^2 + \phi_2^2 r^2\right)}}$$

E8. Q-Switched Nd:YAG Laser.

Consider a Q-Switched Nd:YAG laser (1.064 μm) that has cross-section beam profiles illustrated in Figures E8-1 and E8-2 (profile is marked "raw data"). The beam profile is measured at the back focal plane (infinity focal point) of a 1.9 m focal length lens, designed to focus 1.064 μm laser light with minimal aberrations. The beam path is also shielded to reduce atmospheric effects. The measurement is conducted with a beam profiler and beam image profiles captured for analysis by software methods. These profiler images are provided in Figure E8-3. The energy per pulse is measured to be 85 mJ.

The beam profiles at the back focal plane of the lens (the far-field profiles) are subjected to a variety of laser beam profiling techniques including a "least squares" Gaussian functional fit, ISO 11146 Part 1 analysis, and the measurement of the peak pixel radiant exposure. The resulting analyses, as listed in Table E8-1, indicate that two of the standard methods of beam characterization, the ISO 11146 Part 1 and Gaussian Fits, do agree with one another in terms of divergence, however, they do not accurately capture a value critical for safety assessments: the peak energy emitted per solid angle in the far field. In the cases of the ISO 11146 Part 1 and Gaussian Fit, the peak irradiance emitted per solid angle is approximately 120% of the modeled value for Profile 1. For the Profile 2, the ISO 11146 Part 1 technique overestimates peak irradiance by about 40%, while the Gaussian Fit underestimates the exposure by about 20%. We attribute this to the fact that those methods are weighted by the outlying energy in the profiles acquired, and in the case of the illuminator laser, the profile is somewhat of a "top-hat" function. Because the Peak/Total Energy method is constrained to match the peak energy level, the prediction of maximum exposure is accurate. For these reasons, the Peak/Total Energy method was chosen for purposes of hazard analysis for both profiles of the lasers. The three analysis models agree to within the quoted uncertainties.

Table E8-1. Far Field Beam Profile Analysis Results

Measurement Method	Profile 1 Beam Divergence (μrad)	Profile 2 Beam Divergence (μrad)
ISO 11146 – 4 Sigma ($1/e^2$)	346 ± 24	1140 ± 40
Gaussian Fit ($1/e^2$)	348 ± 34	1470 ± 60
Peak/Total Energy Equivalent Gaussian ($1/e^2$)	318 ± 14	1330 ± 40

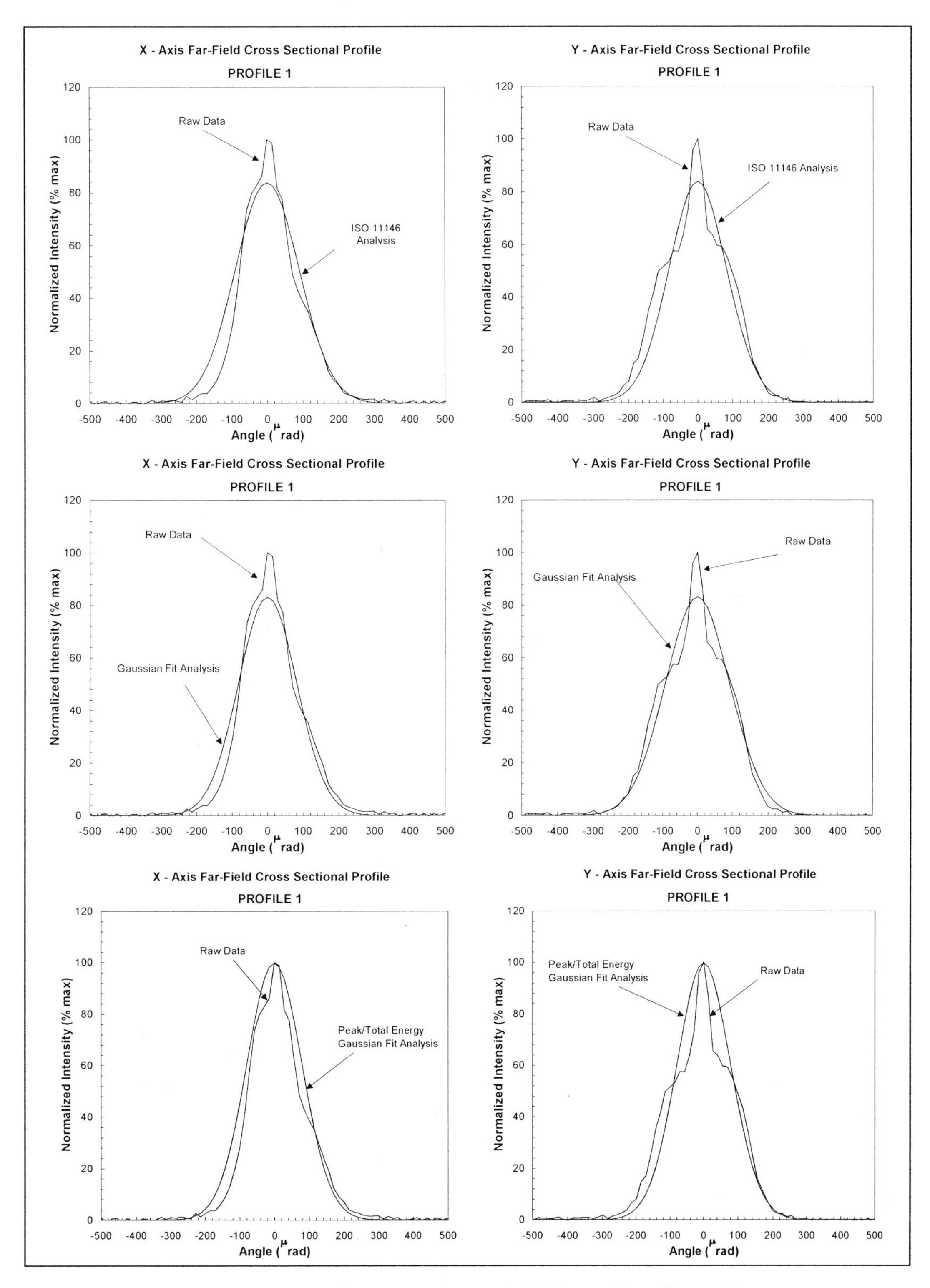

Figure E8-1. Cross Sectional Far-Field Beam Profiles with Corresponding Analysis Results – Profile 1

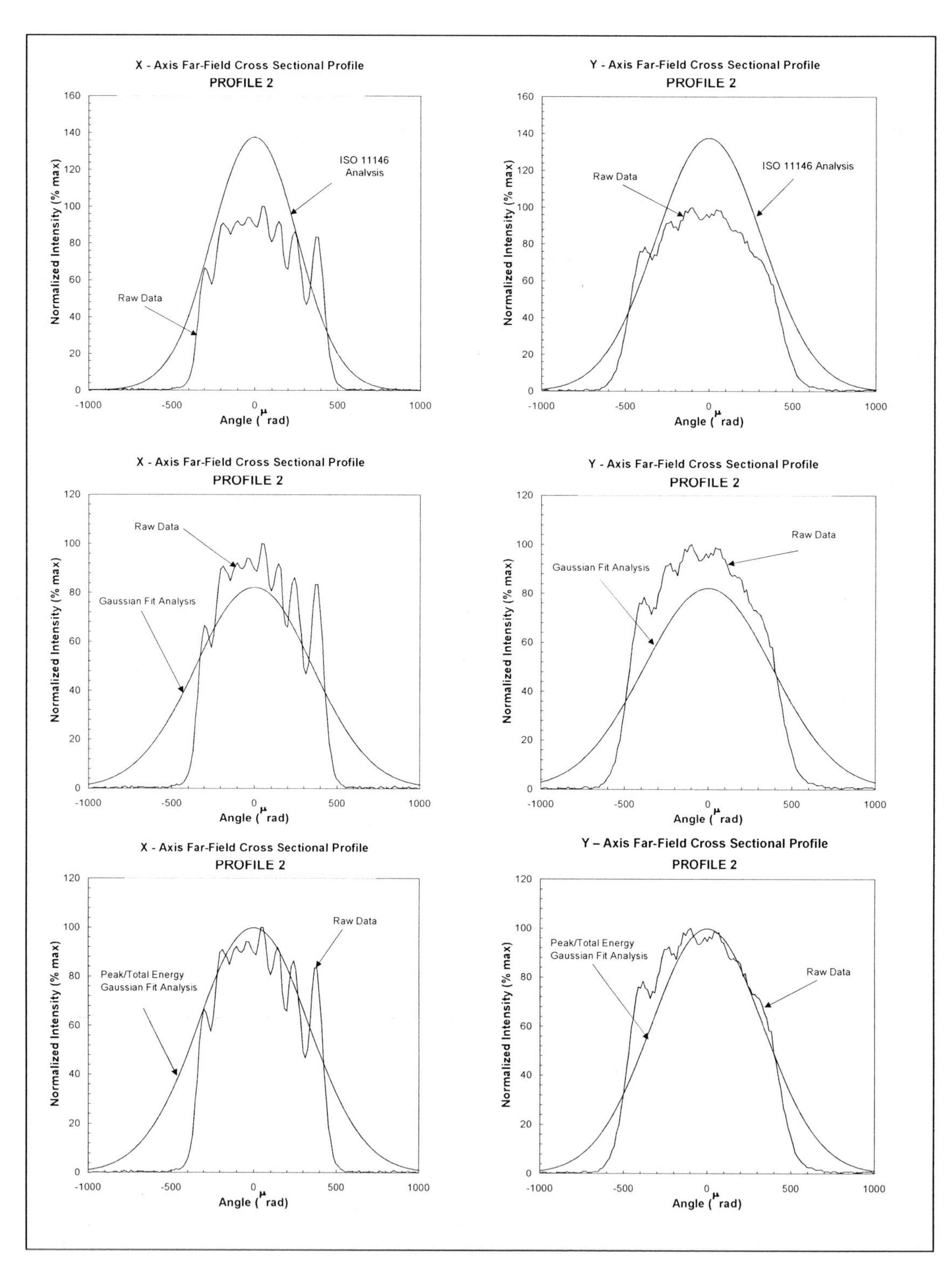

Figure E8-2. Cross Sectional Far-Field Beam Profiles with Corresponding Analysis Results – Profile 2

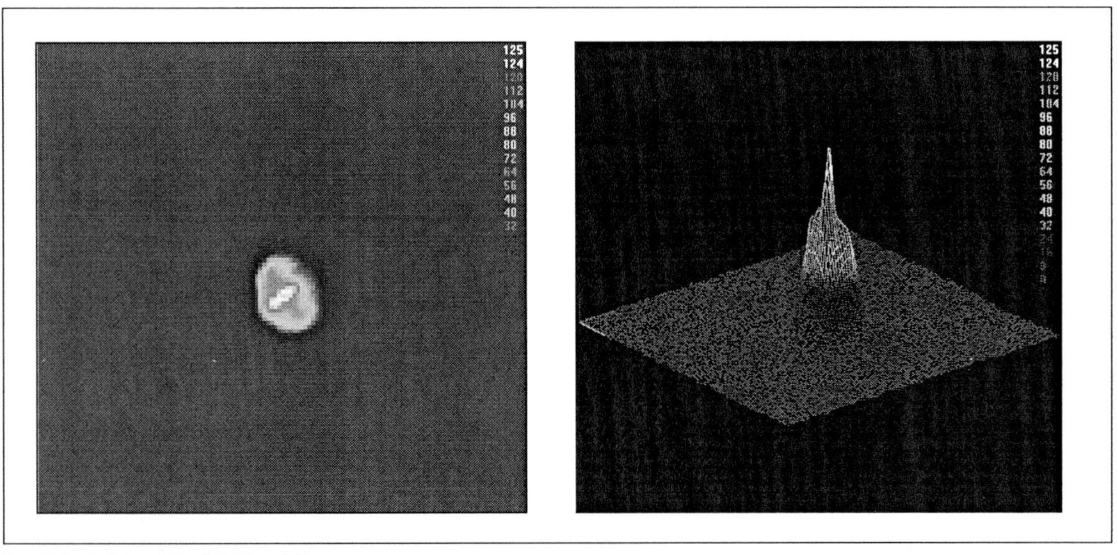

Profile 1 Far Field Profile

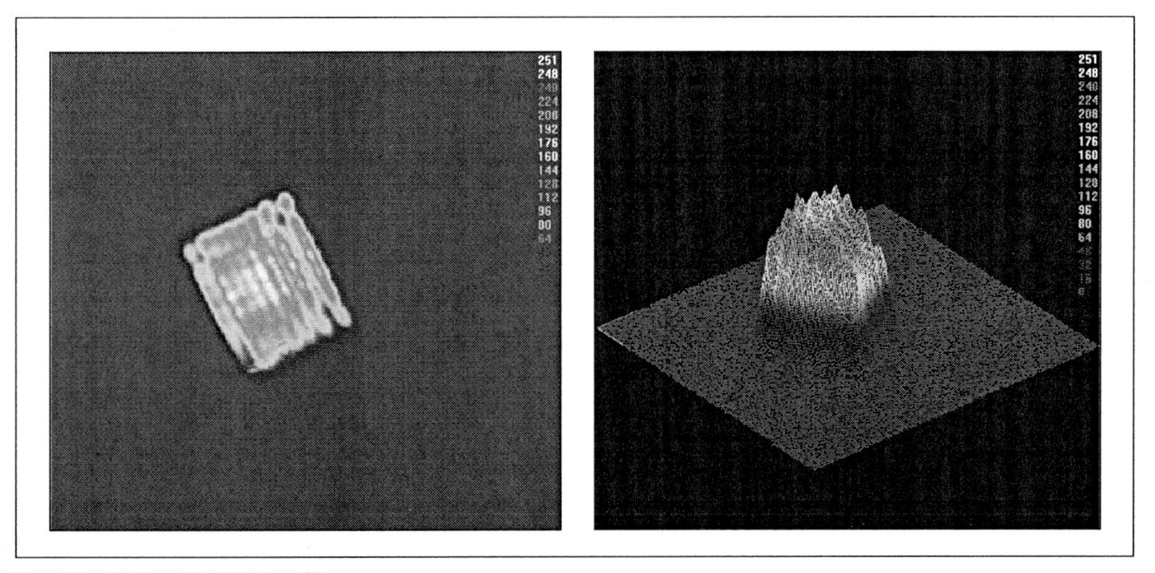

Profile 2 Far Field Profile

Figure E8-3. Far-Field Beam Profiles 1 and 2

E9. Beam Divergence.

A large-aperture, pulsed Nd:YAG laser system has the manufacturer specified output parameters shown in Table E9-1. A measurement of laser beam divergence is required, and equipment is available for several types of measurements, all of which will have to use a lens, with a 3 m focal length, and a clear aperture of 15 cm.

Table E9-1. Laser Beam Parameters for Example 9

Parameter	Value
Pulse Energy	50 mJ
Exit Beam Profile	Gaussian
PRF	20 Hz
Exit Beam Dia. ($1/e^2$) radiant exposure pts.	10 cm
Exit Aperture Dia.	15 cm
Beam Divergence ($1/e^2$) radiant exposure pts.	Unknown
Wavelength	1.064 μm

The lens will be used to collect and focus the beam, the divergence being determined by measuring the size of the beam at the focal length of this lens. The divergence ϕ is computed from the beam size using the equation:

$$\phi = \frac{D_{fs}}{f}$$

where f is the focal length of the lens and D_{fs} is the diameter of the beam at the focal length of the lens. For the purposes of this example, D_{fs} will be measured at the $1/e^2$ radiant exposure point.

We can estimate the minimum beam diameter that may have to be measured at the focal length of the lens by computing the diffraction-limited divergence of the beam. The equation that we need for this is:

$$\phi_{d.l.} \approx \frac{2\lambda}{\pi D_L}$$

$$\phi_{d.l.} \approx \frac{2 \cdot 1.064\ \mu m}{\pi \cdot 10\ \text{cm}}$$

$$\phi_{d.l.} \approx 13\,\mu\text{rad}$$

meaning that the spot size to be measured will have a diameter of approximately 39 μm.

Now we will examine three possible techniques for measuring this small spot diameter in order to determine the beam divergence.

Case 1. CCD camera: A CCD camera with image capture software and image analysis tools can be considered. The typical CCD camera will have an individual pixel width on the order of 10 μm. This means that if the beam is collimated to a nearly diffraction-limited divergence, the beam will be sampled at only about four points across the cross section of the beam, within the

$1/e^2$ diameter. The measurement of spot diameter will therefore be very coarse, and accurate to approximately 20-25%. If it is possible to obtain accurate beam diameter, this technique is often desirable in order to map the radiant exposure distribution profile and apply more detailed analyses found in the ISO 11146 standards.

Case 2. Circular Aperture Measurement: A small pinhole near the focal length of the lens can also be used to measure the spot diameter. A pinhole with a diameter near that of the anticipated 1/e irradiance point diameter is commonly selected. The energy transmitted through the pinhole determines the beam diameter according to the equation:

$$D_L = \sqrt{\frac{-D_{fa}^{2}}{\ln\left(1-\frac{\Phi_d}{\Phi_0}\right)}}$$

The value of D_{fa} is the diameter of the pinhole, Φ_d is the beam energy transmitted through the aperture, and Φ_0 is the output of the laser. In order to obtain an accurate result, the pinhole size should be selected so that the energy transmitted is less than 80% of the total beam and large enough that sufficient energy is transmitted to measure accurately. Because the beam divergence will usually be larger than the diffraction limit, a number of pinholes may be needed to have one with the correct size. Due to the concentration of the beam energy, the pinhole may be enlarged (and burned) due to the high radiant exposure, especially if the laser is Q-switched.

Case 3. Knife-Edge Measurement: A single knife-edge aperture, scanned through the beam can be used to determine the spot size of the laser at the focal length of the lens. As the knife-edge scans through the beam, the fraction of transmitted energy for a Gaussian profile will decrease according to the function:

$$\frac{\Phi_x}{\Phi_0} = 0.5 \times \left[1 + erf\left(\frac{(x - x_0)}{\sqrt{2}\omega}\right)\right]$$

where x is the knife-edge position, x_0 is the center of the beam, and ω is the radius of the beam at the $1/e^2$ irradiance point. The data can be fitted to the above equation, to determine the beam radius. The distance between two points where 14 and 86% of the laser power are transmitted is equal to the radius of the beam at the $1/e^2$ irradiance point, ω. Because a micrometer can be used for this experiment, or a stepper motor scan drive, the measured values can be accurate to a few micrometers. A wide range of spot diameters can also be addressed, making the measurement less sensitive to how nearly diffraction limited the beam is collimated.

Important Note: For the beam parameters specified, a focused beam will have an extremely large peak irradiance value. The beam must be attenuated to below the damage threshold for the pinhole, knife-edge aperture, CCD camera, and detector used in the experiment. This is typically done by reflecting the beam from the front surface of a high-quality, flat wedge prism. The beam can also be attenuated with a neutral density filter or a combination of the two methods. However, introduction of these additional optical elements can significantly affect the results if the components are not of the best quality.

E10. Extended Sources.

Consider the following laser diode collimator-projection system: A visible diode output is collected and transmitted through an optical fiber. The laser system has a 2.1 cm output aperture short focal length lens that collimates the output from the fiber-optic emitter. The fiber tip is located near the focal point of the lens, and has a core diameter of 200 μm. The manufacturer of the laser system wishes to characterize the laser system extended source characteristics and compute the correct MPE value as a function of range from the laser. Describe the measurement of the extended source size as a function of the observer's range and compute the correction to the MPE given the laser parameters listed in Table E10-1 and the sample data provided later in the example in Table E10-2.

Table E10-1. Laser Beam Parameters

Parameter	Value
Average Output Power	22 mW
Exit Beam Profile	Clipped Gaussian
Exit Beam Dia. (1/e) irradiance pts.	1.2 cm
Beam Divergence (1/e) irradiance pts.	4.0 mrad
Wavelength	0.650 μm

A laser diode operating with no external optics widely diverges when compared with solid-state (Nd:YAG, for example) or gas lasers (Ar, Kr, and HeNe, for example). For most laser diode pointer/illuminators, a short focal length lens is used to collimate the output of the diode laser. The result of this design is to reduce the divergence angle of the beam. The beam, however well collimated, will have a finite divergence angle and the beam diameter will expand with distance due to diffraction.

The emission from the collimated diode laser beam is often designed to produce an image of the laser diode, or in the case of fiber-optic coupling of diode to projection lens, an image of the fiber tip at a distance (either a virtual or real image may be formed). The energy from the laser will not be focused to a diffraction-limited spot at the image distance, but an image of the fiber tip or diode laser face is formed.

When an observer views the emitting source (fiber tip or LED) by looking into the beam (with laser eye protection, or by using a camera), the laser output appears to come from a finite area. This area may appear to be rectangular or several closely spaced rectangles when the diode itself is viewed, or it may appear to be a circular structure in the case of a fiber being used to couple the laser diode output. The apparent visual angle subtended by the source from the perspective of the observer, as shown in the top panel of Figure E10-1, is computed from equation:

$$\alpha_{\text{fiber}}(r) = \frac{D_{\text{fiber}}(r)}{r}$$

based upon the assumption $D_{\text{fiber}} << r$. Here $\alpha_{\text{fiber}}(r)$ is the visual angle subtended, $D_{\text{fiber}}(r)$ is the diameter of the fiber core that an observer sees at a distance ***r***.

The lower panel of Figure E10-1 shows the ray diagram of the emitter source placed inside the focal length *f* of a collimating lens. Figure E10-2 shows the visual angle measurement setup. The distance measured from the back principal plane of the collimating lens to the emitter is labeled ***s***. A virtual image of the emitter is formed far behind the source at a distance *s'*. The resulting angle subtended by this virtual image, in the field of view of an observer, at a range of *R* from the collimating lens is:

$$\alpha(R) = \frac{D_{\text{fiber}} \times f}{fR + fs - sR}.$$

In this convention, the quantities *s'* and α are negative in sign. Also, the apparent source diameter, D_{d}, can then be computed from the magnification *M* and equation:

$$D_{\text{d}} = M \times D_{\text{fiber}} = \frac{f \times D_{\text{fiber}}}{(f - s)}.$$

The magnifying lens has a limited clear aperture and the apparent source size will be limited to that diameter. Beyond a range of $R > D_{\text{exit}} / \alpha_0$ (where α_0 is the angular subtense at the collimating lens) the angle subtended will be limited to:

$$\alpha(R) = \frac{D_{\text{exit}}}{R}$$

In the limit that *s* approaches *f*, the apparent visual angle becomes a constant, equal to the beam divergence.

$$\lim_{s \to f} \alpha(R) = \frac{D_{\text{fiber}}}{f}.$$

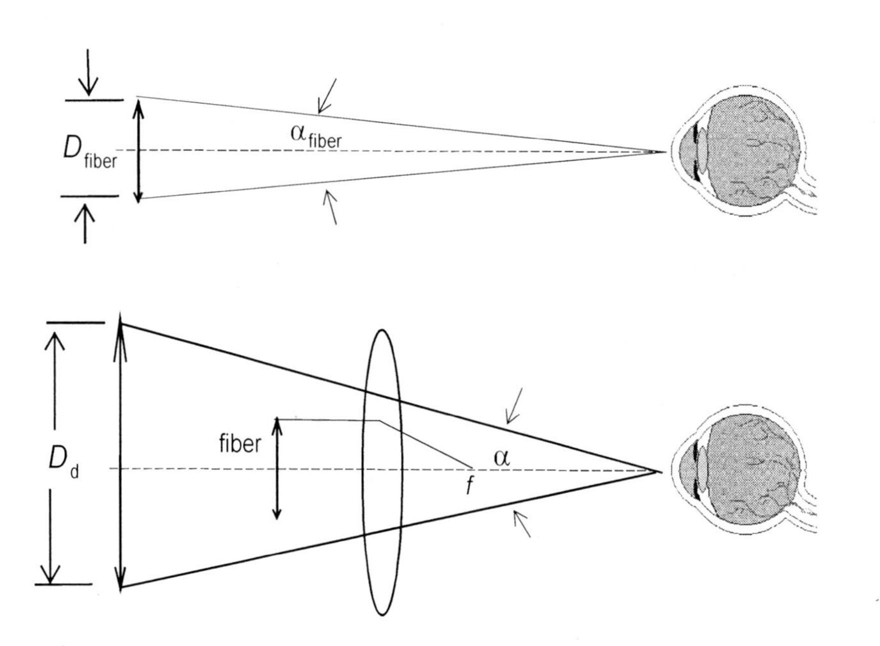

Figure E10-1. Extended Source Ray Diagrams - Laser System Design

Measurement of Visual Angle

The apparent visual angle subtended by an extended source can be measured by imaging the output of the laser diode collimator. By placing a lens of a known focal length f in the beam in place of the observer, and imaging the emitting surface, a real image is formed near (but beyond) the focal length of the lens with an image diameter, D_{image}, at a distance s_m from the lens. The image of the fiber optic exit face subtends an angle with the measurement lens equal to that of the apparent visual angle at the location of the measurement lens. (See Figure E10-2.) The subtended angle is then computed using the equation:

$$\alpha(lens) = \frac{D_{\text{image}}}{s_{\text{m}}}$$

For this method to work, the virtual image of the extended source must be farther from the lens than its focal length, and the lens must have sufficient resolving power to image the emitting surface. The apparent visual angle at locations, other than the location of the measurement lens, will vary unless the diode laser is extremely well collimated.

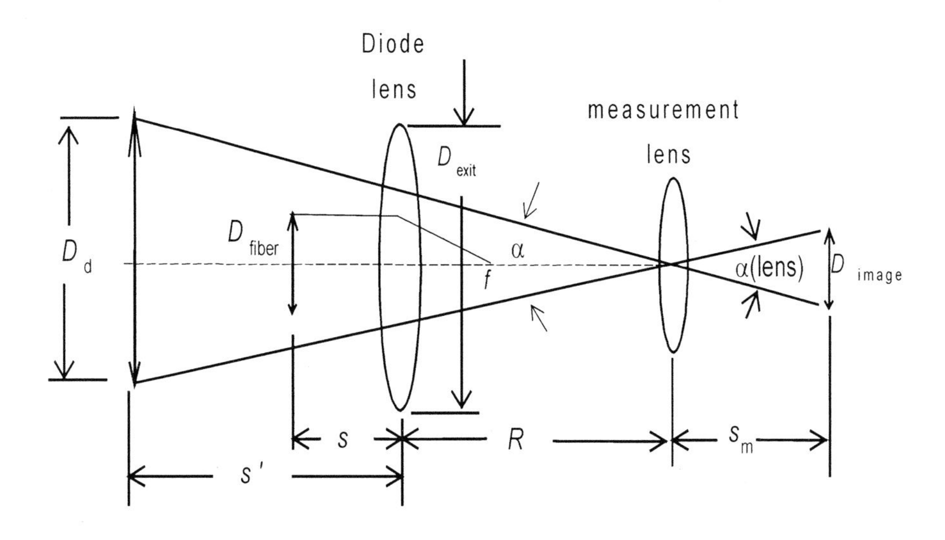

Figure E10-2. Visual Angle Measurement Setup

Measurement Data

Measurements are performed on the laser unit, of subtended visual angle as a function of range, tabulated between 1 m and 6 m from the laser output aperture using a 250 mm focal length lens with a 48 mm clear aperture. Images are captured and analyzed using a CCD camera laser beam profiling system. Image size is determined by measuring the full-width at half-maximum of the imaged fiber. An uncertainty in measurement of 4 pixels is estimated. This yields an uncertainty of ±0.22 mrad in visual angle subtended. Resulting data values are listed in Table E10-2.

Table E10-2. Visual Angle Measurements

Range (m)	Image Size (µm) [full width, half maximum]	Visual Angle (mrad)	C_E
1	702 ± 54	2.81 ± 0.22	1.87 ± 0.15
2	486 ± 54	1.94 ± 0.22	1.29 ± 0.15
3	405 ± 54	1.62 ± 0.22	1.08 ± 0.15
4	393 ± 54	1.57 ± 0.22	1.05 ± 0.15
5	351 ± 54	1.40 ± 0.22	--
6	297 ± 54	1.19 ± 0.22	--

The visual angle subtended by the laser can be computed as a function of range if the values for f, s, and D_{fiber} are known. The specifications for the laser indicate that the fiber diameter is 200 µm. The value of s and f are determined from the lens data and laser design specifications to be 49.4 mm, and 50.2 mm respectively. Figure E10-3 illustrates the resulting visual angle $\alpha(R)$ computed using the equation:

$$\alpha(R) = \frac{D_{\text{fiber}} \times f}{fR + fs - sR}.$$

The dashed line in the figure represents values of $\alpha(R)$ determined from an average value of ***s*** computed from the measured values of $\alpha(R)$. This average value produces 49.1 mm for ***s***, compared with the 49.4 mm determined from design and manufacturer specifications.

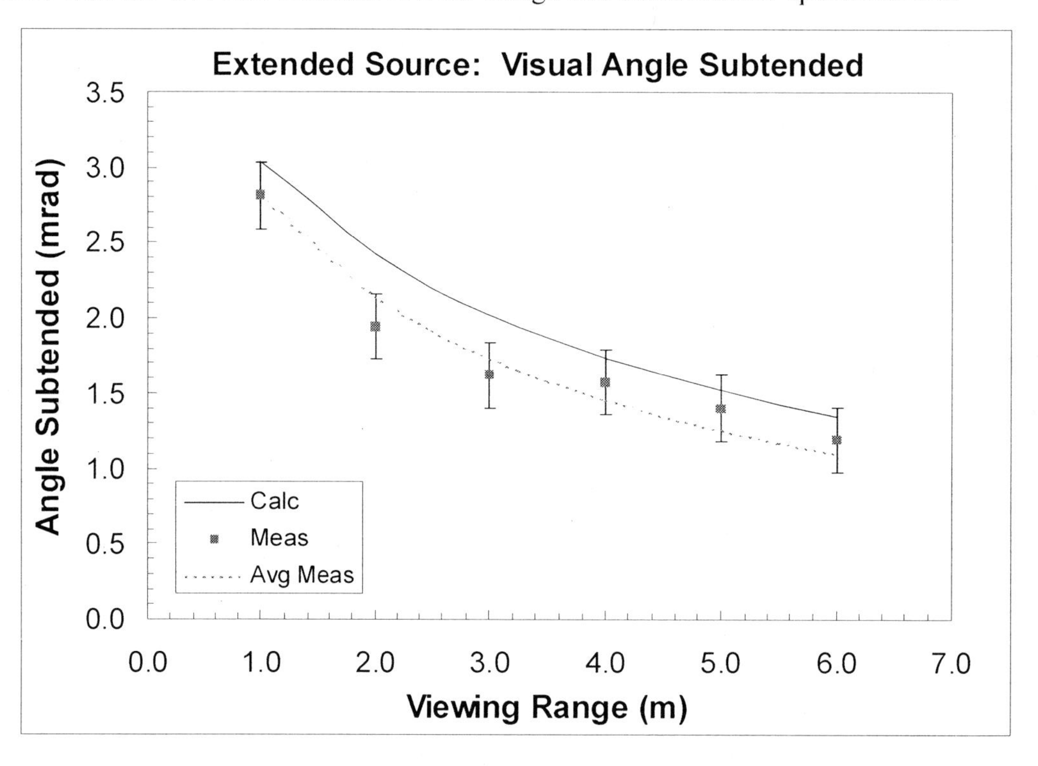

Figure E10-3. Extended Source Size Measurements and Computations

Permissible Exposures (ANSI Z136.1-2007)

The ANSI Standard (ANSI Z136.1-2007), Tables 5a and 5b, establish the MPE for the laser (CW output, 650 nm) equal to:

$$MPE = (1.8t^{3/4} \times 10^{-3}\,\text{J/cm}^2)/t$$

for a point source, which for an exposure of t=0.25 s, becomes 2.55 mW·cm^{-2}.

The ANSI standard states in Section 8.1 that for exposures of a few seconds, an extended source correction factor is applied to the point-source MPE:

$$MPE = C_{\text{E}} \times MPE_{\text{point-source}}$$

The corrected MPE is used for lasers made from diode arrays or large laser diodes, and for exposure to laser energy reflected from diffusely reflecting surfaces. The distinction between a point source and an extended source for intrabeam viewing is determined from the apparent visual angle of the emitting source as seen by an observer looking at the laser source from within the beam. For the laser system a source angle greater than 1.5 mrad at the observer's location would qualify the system as an extended source and modify the MPE by the extended source correction factor C_E, which is equal to α/α_{min} for angles between 1.5 mrad and 100 mrad. Here, α is the visual angle subtended by the source and α_{min} is 1.5 mrad. The extended source criterion is therefore met at distances up to this range. Beyond this range, we apply the small-source (or point-source) MPE (C_E = 1). Figure E10-4 depicts a comparison of the various MPEs. On this graph, the beam irradiance in the laser beam is shown, dropping below the small-source MPE at approximately 6 m. The laser irradiance is above both the "calculated" and "measured" MPEs at all ranges within 6 m.

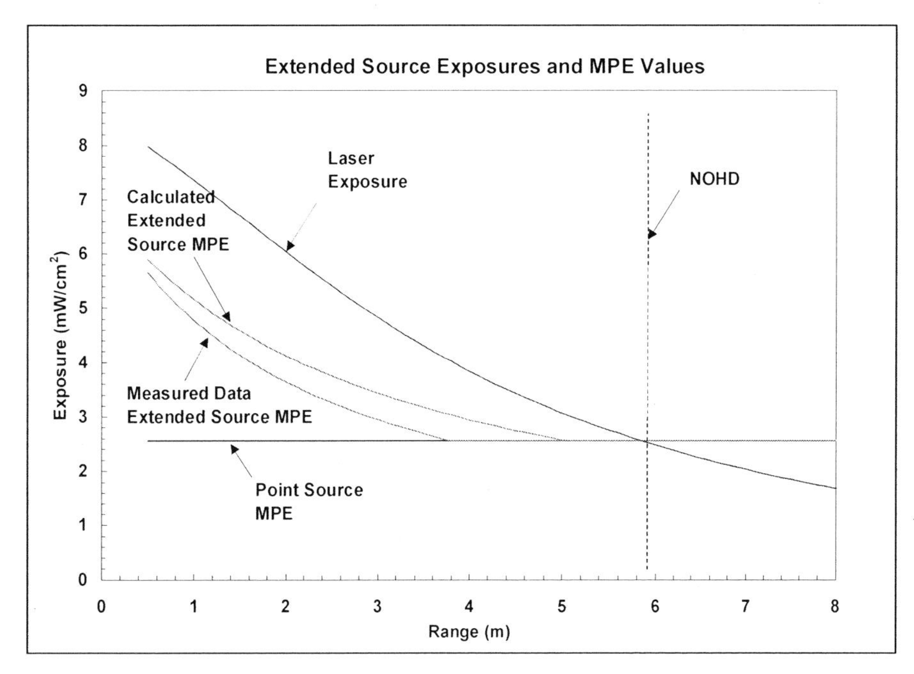

Figure E10-4. Laser Beam Irradiance and MPE Comparison

E11. Uncertainty Analysis.

An example is presented to clarify the application of uncertainty analysis to laser data and results. The approach presented here follows the document *NIST Technical Note 1297, 1994 Edition: Guidelines for Evaluating and Expressing the Uncertainty of NIST Measurement Results*. A brief overview of uncertainty analysis is followed by its application to four examples: (1) determination of pulse energy, (2) determination of maximum permissible exposure (MPE), (3) determination of nominal ocular hazard distance (NOHD), and (4) determination of optical density (OD) required at the exit aperture.

In general, the result of a measurement y is an estimate of the value of the specific quantity subject to measurement, the measurand Y. The result y is obtained from n other estimated quantities x_i through the functional relationship f, given by

$$y = f(x_1, x_2, \ldots, x_i, \ldots, x_n) \ . \tag{11-1}$$

The standard uncertainty of an input quantity x_i is the estimated standard deviation associated with this quantity and is denoted by $u(x_i)$. The estimated standard uncertainty in the measurand y is the combined standard uncertainty $u_c(y)$, given by the law of propagation of uncertainty as

$$u_c^2(y) = \sum_{i=1}^{n} \left(\frac{\partial f}{\partial x_i} \right)^2 u^2(x_i) + 2 \sum_{i=1}^{n-1} \sum_{j=i+1}^{n} \left(\frac{\partial f}{\partial x_i} \right) \left(\frac{\partial f}{\partial x_j} \right) \cdot u(x_i, x_j) \ . \tag{11-2}$$

Here, $\partial f / \partial x_i$ is the sensitivity coefficient with respect to x_i and $u(x_i, x_j)$ is the covariance of x_i and x_j. While the covariance can play an important role in some uncertainty analyses, it has no application for the examples presented here since the uncertainties are uncorrelated. Therefore, the covariance is omitted in the following, so Eq. (11-2) becomes

$$u_c^2(y) = \sum_{i=1}^{n} \left(\frac{\partial f}{\partial x_i} \right)^2 u^2(x_i) \ . \tag{11-3}$$

It is often more convenient to use relative standard uncertainties, $u(x_i)/x_i$, instead of standard uncertainties. Dividing by y^2 and re-arranging, Eq. (11-3) becomes

$$\frac{u_c^2(y)}{y^2} = \sum_{i=1}^{n} \left(\frac{x_i}{y} \frac{\partial f}{\partial x_i} \right)^2 \frac{u^2(x_i)}{x_i^2} \ , \tag{11-4}$$

in which the relative standard and combined uncertainties are used and the relative sensitivity coefficient is given by (x_i/y) $(\partial f / \partial x_i)$. Equation (11-4) is useful for most applications in laser safety measurements, in which the functional relationship is multiplicative, for example Eqs. (11-5), (11-7), and (11-9) below.

The four examples of uncertainty calculations are all based on a pulsed laser with nominal characteristics of wavelength $\lambda = 807$ nm, pulse energy $Q = 2$ mJ, pulse duration $t = 20$ µs, and pulse-repetition-frequency $PRF = 13$ kHz. The four example uncertainty calculations using this laser illustrate the progression of uncertainties from a measure of pulse energy to the safety aspects of the nominal ocular hazard distance and laser eye protection optical density.

The examples also attempt to follow the rules for significant figures, although this topic as it applies to uncertainty calculations is beyond the scope of this appendix. Most input quantity values have three significant figures, while provided uncertainties, either standard or relative standard, have one significant figure. Calculations of uncertainties usually have two significant figures, in order to be able to reproduce the provided uncertainties, and the final combined uncertainty has as many decimal places as the value of the result. The value of the result usually has three significant figures, which determines the number of decimal places of the combined uncertainty.

The pulse energy of the laser is measured using a calibrated joulemeter, lens, and wedge prism. The functional relationship between the result, pulse energy Q, and the input parameters is

$$Q = S \times C \times \tau \times \rho \ , \qquad (11\text{-}5)$$

where S [V] is the signal measured by the joulemeter, C [$mJ \cdot V^{-1}$] is the manufacturer calibration relating the signal to the pulse energy, τ is the transmittance of the lens, and ρ is the reflectance of the wedge prism. The values for these input quantities, as well as their standard uncertainties, are given in Table E11-1.

Table E11-1. Standard Uncertainties and Combined Uncertainty for the Pulse Energy Measurement Example

Input Quantity x_i	Value	Std. Unc. $u(x_i)$	Unit	Type	Rel. Std. Uncertainty $u(x_i)/x_i$ [%]	Rel. Sens. Coefficient $(x_i/y)(\partial f/\partial x_i)$	Uncertainty Contribution $u_i(y)/y$ [%]
Signal, S	2.04	0.07	V	A	3.4	1	3.4
Calibration, C	27.5	1.4	$mJ \cdot V^{-1}$	B	5	1	5
Transmittance, τ	0.907	0.005	---	B	0.5	1	0.5
Reflectance, ρ	0.0431	0.0001	---	B	0.2	1	0.2
Result y	Value	Comb. Unc. $u_c(y)$	Unit				Rel. Comb. Uncertainty $u_c(y)/y$ [%]
Pulse Energy, Q	2.19	0.13	mJ				6.1

This table requires detailed explanation, as it includes important concepts for uncertainty analyses. The upper portion contains information and results about the input quantities, while the lower portion contains the results from the uncertainty analysis for the measurement result. For the upper portion, the first column lists the input quantities, as given by Eq. (11-5). The second column lists the values for these input quantities, as obtained from measurements or other sources, and the fourth column lists the units for these quantities. In this example, the value for the signal is the average of multiple readings of the joulemeter, while the other values are obtained from the calibration certificates for these items.

The third column lists the standard uncertainty for each input quantity, while the sixth column lists the relative standard uncertainty. Typically, either the standard uncertainty or relative standard uncertainty is calculated or provided, and the other is derived from it. In this example, the value for the signal is the average of multiple readings of the joulemeter, and the standard uncertainty is the standard deviation of the mean of the multiple readings. The relative standard uncertainty is then simply the standard uncertainty divided by the value. In contrast, the relative standard uncertainties for the other input quantities are supplied with the calibration certificates for these items, and the standard uncertainties are calculated from these and the values. For example, the joulemeter calibration certificate reports a value of 27.5 $mJ \cdot V^{-1}$ with a relative standard uncertainty of 5%, resulting in a standard uncertainty of 1.4 $mJ \cdot V^{-1}$. The fifth column lists the type of uncertainty evaluation used to obtain the standard uncertainties. Type A evaluations use statistical methods, while Type B evaluations use other methods. Since the standard uncertainty for the joulemeter signal was obtained from the standard deviation of the mean, its Type is A. The other standard uncertainties were obtained from the calibration certificates, and so are Type B.

The seventh column lists the relative sensitivity coefficients, obtained by performing the indicated operation on Eq. (11-5) for each input quantity. In this example, since Eq. (11-5) is a simple multiplication of input quantities, the relative sensitivity coefficients are trivial. Subsequent examples will have more complicated entries in this column. From Eq. (11-4), the relative uncertainty contribution of each input quantity on the final result is obtained by multiplying the relative sensitivity coefficient (seventh column) by the relative standard uncertainty (sixth column), and the results of these calculations are listed in the eighth column.

The lower portion of the table contains the resulting uncertainty for the pulse energy. As for the upper portion, the first, second, and fourth columns list the result, value, and unit. The value is obtained by substituting the values in the second column of the upper portion into Eq. (11-5). The eighth column lists the relative combined uncertainty, obtained using Eq. (11-4) by summing the squares of the values in the eighth column of the upper portion of the table and taking the square root of the result (i.e., $6.1 = [3.4^2 + 5^2 + 0.4^2 + 0.2^2]^{1/2}$). Finally, the third column lists the resulting combined uncertainty, obtained by multiplying the relative combined uncertainty by the value of the result. Here, 6.1% of 2.19 mJ is 0.13 mJ. Note that the combined uncertainty could be obtained directly from the standard uncertainties, using Eq. (11-3); the process of converting to relative standard and combined uncertainties and using relative sensitivity coefficients is for ease of calculation and gives an indication of the relative contributions of each input quantity, from the eighth column, to the combined uncertainty. In this example, the two primary contributors are the joulemeter signal and calibration.

One additional consideration for uncertainty analyses not shown in the table, but which is important, is the concept of expanded uncertainty U, given by

$$U = k \times u_c(y) \ , \qquad (11\text{-}6)$$

where k is the coverage factor. The expanded uncertainty defines an interval about the result y within which the measurand Y lies with a given level of confidence. For a normal probability distribution, this level of confidence is 68.2% for $k = 1$ and 95.45% for $k = 2$. For most applications, a coverage factor of 2 is used. Completing the example, the pulse energy would be reported as $Q = 2.19 \pm 0.26$ mJ, with a coverage factor $k = 2$.

While much detail was given for a relatively simple uncertainty analysis of pulse energy, the concepts and techniques will prove useful when considering the more complicated problems of uncertainty analyses for MPE, NOHD, and OD.

The wavelength λ, pulse-repetition-frequency PRF, and pulse duration t of the pulsed laser are all measured, and their standard uncertainties determined. The results are $\lambda = 807 \pm 1$ nm, $PRF = 13.139 \pm 0.066$ kHz, and $t = 19.6 \pm 0.2$ μs. Since the laser is pulsed, the three-rule method for repeated exposures must be used to determine the MPE. An exposure time $T = 10$ s is used in the calculations of the three-rule method. The resulting MPEs are 8.68×10^{-7} J·cm^{-2}, 1.25×10^{-7} J·cm^{-2}, and 4.56×10^{-8} J·cm^{-2} for the three rules, respectively, so the MPE for the third rule is applicable. The single-pulse MPE for this wavelength and pulse duration is given by

$$MPE_{\mathrm{p}} = 1.8 \times C_{\mathrm{A}} \times t^{0.75} \times 10^{-3}\ \mathrm{J{\cdot}cm^{-2}}, \quad (11\text{-}7)$$

where

$$C_{\mathrm{A}} = 10^{2(\lambda - 0.700)}\ . \quad (11\text{-}8)$$

Note that the unit for wavelength in Eq. (11-8) is μm. The multiple-pulse MPE for thermal hazards is the applicable one for this laser, given by

$$MPE = \left(n_{\mathrm{eff}}\right)^{-0.25} \times MPE_{\mathrm{p}}\ , \quad (11\text{-}9)$$

where

$$n_{\mathrm{eff}} = PRF \times T \quad (11\text{-}10)$$

and the dependence on k in Eqs. (11-9) and (11-10) has been omitted since $k = 1$. Given the number and complexity of equations necessary to determine the MPE, the uncertainty analysis for the MPE appears to be a daunting task. However, applying the approach illustrated by Table E11-1, the uncertainty in MPE can be obtained by dividing the problem into tractable parts.

From Eq. (11-9), the uncertainty in MPE depends upon the uncertainties in n_{eff} and MPE_{p}. The former, from Eq. (11-10), depends upon the uncertainties in PRF and T. The latter, from Eq. (11-7), depends upon the uncertainties in C_{A} and t, and from Eq. (11-8) the uncertainty in C_{A} depends upon the uncertainty in λ. Working backwards from the progression just given, tables equivalent to Table E11-1 are constructed for the uncertainties in C_{A}, MPE_{p}, and n_{eff}, and these are the inputs for a final table for the uncertainty in MPE. In particular, the result from Table E11-2 is an input for Table E11-3, and the results from Tables E11-3 and E11-4 are inputs for Table E11-5. The equations used to obtain the relative sensitivity coefficients for each table are indicated in the notes. The combined uncertainty for the MPE, given in Table E11-5, is the result of the measured uncertainties for the wavelength, PRF, and pulse duration.

Table E11-2. Standard Uncertainties and Combined Uncertainty for Correction Factor C_{A} for the MPE Example

Input Quantity x_i	Value	Std. Unc. $u(x_i)$	Unit	Type	Rel. Std. Uncertainty $u(x_i)/x_i$ [%]	Rel. Sens. Coefficient $(x_i/y)(\partial f/\partial x_i)$	Uncertainty Contribution $u_i(y)/y$ [%]
Wavelength, λ	807	1	nm	A	0.12	$4.6 \times 10^{-3} \times \lambda$*	0.44
Result y	Value	Comb. Unc. $u_c(y)$	Unit				Rel. Comb. Uncertainty $u_c(y)/y$ [%]
Corr. Fact., C_{A}	1.64	0.01	—				0.44

Note: Eq. (11-8) was used to calculate the relative sensitivity coefficient.

* The wavelength for the relative sensitivity coefficient calculation must be in units of nm.

Table E11-3. Standard Uncertainties and Combined Uncertainty for Single Pulse *MPE*p for the MPE Example

Input Quantity x_i	Value	Std. Unc. $u(x_i)$	Unit	Type	Rel. Std. Uncertainty $u(x_i)/x_i$ [%]	Rel. Sens. Coefficient $(x_i/y)(\partial f/\partial x_i)$	Uncertainty Contribution $u_i(y)/y$ [%]
Corr. Fact., C_A	1.64	0.01	---	B	0.44	1	0.44
Pulse Dur., t	19.6	0.2	μs	A	1.0	0.75	0.75
Result y	Value	Comb. Unc. $u_c(y)$	Unit				Rel. Comb. Uncertainty $u_c(y)/y$ [%]
Pulse, MPE_p	868	8	$nJ \cdot cm^{-2}$				0.87

Note: Eq. (11-7) was used to calculate the relative sensitivity coefficients.

Table E11-4. Standard Uncertainties and Combined Uncertainty for Effective Number of Pulses n_{eff} for the MPE Example

Input Quantity x_i	Value	Std. Unc. $u(x_i)$	Unit	Type	Rel. Std. Uncertainty $u(x_i)/x_i$ [%]	Rel. Sens. Coefficient $(x_i/y)(\partial f/\partial x_i)$	Uncertainty Contribution $u_i(y)/y$ [%]
PRF	13.139	0.066	kHz	A	0.5	1	0.5
Exp. Time, T	10	0*	s	B	0	1	0
Result y	Value	Comb. Unc. $u_c(y)$	Unit				Rel. Comb. Uncertainty $u_c(y)/y$ [%]
Eff. No., n_{eff}	1.3139×10^5	660	---				0.5

Note: Eq. (11-10) was used to calculate the relative sensitivity coefficients.

* The exposure time T is a specified constant, and therefore has no uncertainty

Table E11-5. Standard Uncertainties and Combined Uncertainty for the MPE Example

Input Quantity x_i	Value	Std. Unc. $u(x_i)$	Unit	Type	Rel. Std. Uncertainty $u(x_i)/x_i$ [%]	Rel. Sens. Coefficient $(x_i/y)(\partial f/\partial x_i)$	Uncertainty Contribution $u_i(y)/y$ [%]
Eff. No., n_{eff}	1.3139×10^5	660	---	B	0.5	0.25	0.125
Pulse, MPE_p	868	8	$nJ \cdot cm^{-2}$	B	0.87	1	0.87
Result y	Value	Comb. Unc. $u_c(y)$	Unit				Rel. Comb. Uncertainty $u_c(y)/y$ [%]
Multiple, MPE	45.6	0.4	$nJ \cdot cm^{-2}$				0.88

Note: Eq. (11-9) was used to calculate the relative sensitivity coefficients.

The MPE would be reported as 45.6 ± 0.8 $nJ \cdot cm^{-2}$, with a coverage factor $k = 2$. Note that uncertainties in MPE are dependent on the wavelength and time, as given in Table 5a of the ANSI Z136.1-2007 standard. This pulse laser example was chosen because the MPE depends on both time and wavelength, and therefore illustrates the uncertainty analysis techniques that need to be applied. As an alternative example, the MPE for a laser operating at a wavelength of 1.064 μm with pulse durations between 1 ns and 50 μs does not depend on either the wavelength or the time, and therefore there is no uncertainty associated with this MPE.

The nominal ocular hazard distance, NOHD, in the absence of atmospheric attenuation, is given by

$$\text{NOHD} = \frac{1}{\phi}\sqrt{\frac{4\,Q}{\pi\,MPE} - a^2}\ , \qquad (11\text{-}11)$$

where ϕ is the divergence of the laser beam at the 1/e points and a is the initial diameter of the laser beam at the 1/e points. For this example, these values are all measured, and their standard uncertainties (coverage factor $k = 1$) determined. The results are $\phi = 26.6 \pm 1.4$ mrad and $a = 16.2 \pm 0.6$ cm. The values for Q and MPE, and their uncertainties, are given in Tables E11-1 and E11-5, respectively. The uncertainty contributions and combined uncertainty for the NOHD are given in Table E11-6. The NOHD would be reported as 93 ± 12 m, with a coverage factor $k = 2$.

Table E11-6. Standard Uncertainties and Combined Uncertainty for the NOHD Example

Input Quantity x_i	Value	Std. Unc. $u(x_i)$	Unit	Type	Rel. Std. Uncertainty $u(x_i)/x_i$ [%]	Rel. Sens. Coefficient $(x_i/y)(\partial f/\partial x_i)$ *	Uncertainty Contribution $u_i(y)/y$ [%]
Pulse Energy, Q	2.19	0.13	mJ	B	6.1	$(N^2 \times M)/2$	3.1
MPE	45.6	0.4	$\mathrm{nJ \cdot cm^{-2}}$	B	0.89	$(N^2 \times M)/2$	0.45
Divergence, ϕ	26.6	1.4	mrad	A	5.3	1	5.3
Diameter, a	16.2	0.6	cm	A	3.7	$a^2 \times N^2$	0.016
Result y	Value	Comb. Unc. $u_c(y)$	Unit				Rel. Comb. Uncertainty $u_c(y)/y$ [%]
$NOHD$	93	6	m				6.2

Note: Eq. (11-11) was used to calculate the relative sensitivity coefficients.

$$* \; M = \frac{4\,Q}{\pi\, MPE} = 61{,}149 \text{ cm}^2,\; N = \frac{1}{\phi\, NOHD} = 4.051 \times 10^{-3} \text{ cm}^{-1}$$

Finally, the laser eye protection optical density OD required to safely view the laser beam at the exit aperture is given by

$$\mathrm{OD} = \log_{10}\left(\frac{H}{MPE}\right), \tag{11-12}$$

where H [$\mathrm{J \cdot cm^{-2}}$] is the radiant exposure. The uncertainty in MPE is given in Table E11-5, while the uncertainty in H is determined from uncertainties in pulse energy Q and beam diameter a. Instead of calculating the uncertainty in H from the uncertainties in Q and a, as was done for the previous example, the uncertainties in these quantities are used directly to calculate the uncertainty in OD by substituting the definition of H into Eq. (11-12), with the result

$$\mathrm{OD} = \log_{10}\left(\frac{1}{a^2}\frac{4\,Q}{\pi\, MPE}\right). \tag{11-13}$$

The uncertainties in the input quantities for Eq. (11-13) and the resulting uncertainty in OD are given in Table E11-7. The OD would be reported as 2.37 ± 0.08, with a coverage factor $k = 2$.

Table E11-7. Standard Uncertainties and Combined Uncertainty for the OD Example

Input Quantity x_i	Value	Std. Unc. $u(x_i)$	Unit	Type	Rel. Std. Uncertainty $u(x_i)/x_i$ [%]	Rel. Sens. Coefficient $(x_i/y)(\partial f/\partial x_i)$	Uncertainty Contribution $u_i(y)/y$ [%]
Pulse Energy, Q	2.19	0.13	mJ	B	6.1	0.4343/*OD*	1.1
MPE	45.6	0.4	nJ·cm^{-2}	B	0.89	0.4343/*OD*	0.16
Diameter, a	16.2	0.6	cm	B	3.7	0.8686/*OD*	1.4
Result y	Value	Comb. Unc. $u_c(y)$	Unit				Rel. Comb. Uncertainty $u_c(y)/y$ [%]
OD	2.37	0.04	---				1.8

Note: Eq. (11-13) was used to calculate the relative sensitivity coefficients.

The concepts and techniques of uncertainty analysis, as applied in this example for a pulsed laser, are generally applicable to laser measurements. More advanced topics, such as probability distributions and degrees of freedom, were not discussed but may be important for certain uncertainty analyses. The tables presented for this example are useful for performing an uncertainty analysis in a systematic manner and communicating the inputs and results compactly yet completely.

E12. Beam Splitters.

Laser power measurement using an optical beamsplitter.

Optical beamsplitters are often useful when measuring laser beam power or energy. Using the laser source of Example 1 (a pulsed Nd:YAG laser emits 25 W of average power at 1.064 μm), establish a beamsplitter-based measurement system for measuring beam power and calibration of other detectors of interest.

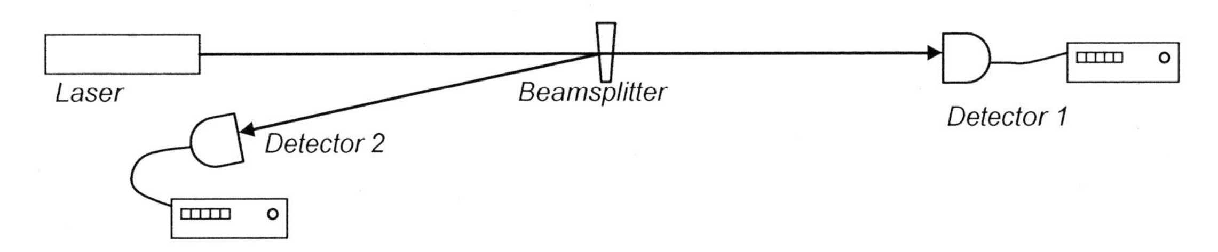

Figure E12-1. Basic Beamsplitter-based Measurement System

The diagram in Figure E12-1 shows a basic beamsplitter-based system in which detectors are placed in the main transmitted beam and the reflected beam from the front surface of the beamsplitter. Any two beams coming from the beamsplitter could be used. Beams not being used should be blocked to prevent stray light from getting to the detectors. For these measurements at 1.064 μm, fused silica (SiO_2), which is highly transparent and has a refractive index of approximately 1.45 at this wavelength, makes a good choice. To prevent interference from the coherent light, the beamsplitter should be wedged, with 2° being a commonly used wedge angle. The ratios of powers (or energies) in the various beams will vary if the polarization is not constant; consequently, to minimize this polarization error (since we do not know for sure whether the polarization is constant for this laser) a small angle of incidence should be used. A small angle of incidence also minimizes errors in case the laser or beamsplitter is accidentally moved during or after the calibration of the beamsplitter. Unfortunately, small angles of incidence also require longer beam paths to allow room for the detectors; consequently, a compromise must usually be made between available space and small angles of incidence.

To use the beamsplitter for quantitative measurements, we want to know the ratio of powers (or energies) in the two beams of interest; consequently, we need to calibrate the beamsplitter. One method of performing this calibration is a three-step procedure as follows:

1. Using the arrangement shown in Figure E12-1 with the laser on and the detectors properly set up, perform a series of measurements in which the output readings of Detectors 1 and 2 are recorded in pairs at about the same time (Note: the readings can be in any units, such as volts, watts, amperes, and joules.). For each pair, the Detector 1 reading is divided by the output reading of Detector 2. Then calculate the average ratio R1 for these runs.
2. Interchange the detectors so that Detector 2 is now in the transmitted beam and Detector 1 is in the reflected beam. Again, perform a series of measurements in which the output readings of the two detectors are recorded in pairs. Now divide the reading of Detector 2 by the reading of Detector 1 for each pair of readings. Then calculate the average ratio R2 for these runs.
3. The beamsplitter ratio R for these two beams is then estimated by calculating the geometric mean of the average ratios $R1$ and $R2$:

$$R = \sqrt{R1 \cdot R2}.$$

In this procedure, detector calibration offsets cancel, so the detectors do not have to be calibrated. However, the detectors need to be linear and spatially uniform since these errors do not cancel in this interchange process. Once the beamsplitter ratio has been determined for the two beams to be used, then the power (or energy) in one beam can be determined by placing a calibrated detector in the other beam. This beamsplitter ratio normally does not vary with power or energy unless some physical change (thermally induced physical distortion) occurs to the beamsplitter material.

Assume that we have performed the steps listed above and obtained the following results:

1. Determine $R1$:

Run #	Detector 1	Detector 2	Ratio
1	22.11	0.83	26.64
2	19.74	0.72	27.42
3	21.92	0.81	27.06
4	18.77	0.7	26.81
5	20.88	0.77	27.12

$R1 = 27.01$ (average of "Ratio" column)

2. Determine $R2$:

Run #	Detector 2	Detector 1	Ratio
1	22.88	0.81	28.25
2	19.74	0.69	28.61
3	21.92	0.79	27.75
4	18.77	0.65	28.88
5	19.98	0.71	28.14

$R2 = 28.33$ (average of "Ratio" column)

3. Determine R:

$$R = \sqrt{R1 \cdot R2} = \sqrt{27.01 \cdot 28.33} = 27.66$$

This ratio is then valid for the detector arrangement used in this calibration. If the polarization changes or the beamsplitter is moved (reoriented) with respect to the laser beam, thus causing a change in the angle of incidence, then a new ratio should be determined.

Now that the beamsplitter is calibrated, let us use a detector from Example E1 (which has previously been calibrated) to measure the power in the main transmitted beam. Place the detector in the reflected beam (where Detector 2 is shown in Figure E12-1) and measure the average power. Then multiply this value by the beamsplitter ratio R to get the average power in the transmitted beam. For example, if the detector in the reflected beam measures 500 mW of average power, then the main transmitted beam has $0.5 \cdot 28 = 14$ W of power. Knowing this, a detector could be placed in the transmitted beam and calibrated by comparing its reading to the actual incident power. If the detector was placed in the transmitted beam, then the average power in the reflected beam could be determined by dividing the meter reading by the beamsplitter ratio. Since the beamsplitter ratio is 28, this, in effect, extends the range of a detector by a factor of 28 higher and lower than its inherent power or energy limits. In this case, the meter only had to be placed in a 500 mW beam to measure 14 W of power. If the beamsplitter is kept clean, then the beamsplitter ratios (especially for uncoated materials) show very little aging, and, thus, the ratios can remain constant for long times (as long as the measurement configuration is not changed).

Appendix F
References

Barat, K., *Laser Safety – Tools & Training*, CRC Press 2009.

Bass, M., Optical Society of America, *Handbook of Optics*, *Vol. I*, McGraw Hill, Inc., New York; 1995.

Budde, W., *Optical Radiation Measurements, Volume 4, Physical Detectors of Optical Radiation*, Academic Press, New York; 1983.

Dereniak, E.L., Crowe D.G. *Optical Radiation Detectors*, John Wiley & Sons, New York; 1984.

Derrick, P., Photon Inc., The Misunderstood M^2 - Understanding the Measurement and Following Proper Procedure Will Yield Accurate Results, Page 30, *SPIE's* OEmagazine; August 2005.

Henderson, R., Schulmeister, K., *Laser Safety*, Institute of Physics Publishing, London; 2004.

Johnston, Jr., T., Beam propagation (M^2) Measurement Made as Easy as It Gets: the Four-cuts Method, Applied Optics, Vol. 37, No. 21; 20 July 1998.

Jones, R.D., Scott, T.R., Laser-Beam Analysis Pinpoints Critical Parameters, *Laser Focus World*, 29(1), 123-130; 1993.

Lyon, T.L., Hazard Analysis Technique for Multiple Wavelength Lasers, Health Physics 49: 221-226; 1985.

Marshall, W.J., Hazard Analysis of Gaussian Shaped Laser Beams, *Am. Ind. Hyg. Assoc. J.* 41, 547-551; 1980.

Marshall, W.J., Conner, P.W., Field Laser Hazard Calculations, *Health Phys.* 52(1), 27-37; 1987.

Marshall, W.J., Determining Hazard Distances from Non-Gaussian Lasers, *Appl. Opt.* 30, 696-698; 1991.

Marshall, W.J., Understanding Laser Hazard Evaluation, *J. Laser Appl.* 7(2), 99-105; 1995.

Marshall, W.J., Aldrich, R.C., Zimmerman, S.A., Laser Hazard Evaluation Method for Middle Infrared Laser Systems, *Journal of Laser Applications* 8: 211-216; 1996.

Marshall, W.J., Determining Source Size from Diode Laser Systems, *Journal of Laser Applications* 14: 252-259; 2002.

Rockwell, B.A., Cain, C.P., Roach, W.P., Thomas, R.J., Safe Use of Ultrashort Lasers. Commercial and Biomedical Applications of Ultrafast Lasers 3616: 32-39; 1999.

Sasnett, M.W., Johnston, Jr., T.F., Beam Characterization and Measurement of Propagation Attributes, *Proc. SPIE*, Vol. 1414 Laser Beam Diagnostics; 1991.

Sliney, D.H., Marshall, W.J., Laser Safety Part IV: Measuring the Beam Diameter, *Electro-Opt. Syst. Design*. 11, 31-36; 1979.

Sliney, D.H., Wolbarsht, M.L., *Safety with Lasers and Other Optical Sources*, Plenum, New York, Third Printing; 1982.

Sliney, D.H., Palmisano, W.A., The Evaluation of Laser Hazards. *American Industrial Hygiene Association Journal* 29: 425-431; 1968.

Taylor, B.N., Kuyatt, C.E., Guidelines for Evaluating and Expressing the Uncertainty of NIST Measurement Results, Natl. Inst. of Stand. Technol., Technical Note 1297; 1994.

Thomas, R.J., Rockwell, B.A., Marshall, W.J., Aldrich, R.C., Gorschboth, M.F., Zimmerman, S.A., Rockwell, R.J., Procedure for the Computation of Hazards from Diffusely Scattering Surfaces under the Z136.1-2000 *American National Standard for Safe Use of Lasers. Journal of Laser Applications* 19: 46-54; 2007.

Thomas, R.J., Rockwell, B.A., Marshall, W.J., Aldrich, R.C., Gorschboth, M.F., Zimmerman, S.A., Rockwell, R.J., A Procedure for the Estimation of Intrabeam Hazard Distances and Optical Density Requirements under the ANSI Z136.1-2000 Standard. *Journal of Laser Applications* 16: 167-177; 2004.

Thomas, R.J., Rockwell, B.A., Marshall, W.J., Aldrich, R.C., Zimmerman, S.A., Rockwell, R.J., A Procedure for Multiple-pulse Maximum Permissible Exposure Determination under the Z136.1-2000 *American National Standard for Safe Use of Lasers. Journal of Laser Applications* 13: 134-140; 2001.

Thomas, R.J., Rockwell, B.A., Marshall, W.J., Aldrich, R.C., Zimmerman, S.A., Rockwell, R.J., A Procedure for Laser Hazard Classification under the Z136.1-2000 *American National Standard for Safe Use of Lasers. Journal of Laser Applications* 14: 57-66; 2002.

Wolfe, W.L., Zissis, G.J., *The Infrared Handbook*, Environmental Research Institute of Michigan; 1989.

Young, M., *Optics and Lasers, 4th Edition*, Springer-Verlag, New York; 1993.

ANSI / IESNA RP-27.1-2005, *Recommended Practice for Photobiological Safety for Lamps and Lamp Systems - General Requirements*

ANSI / IESNA RP-27.2-2000, *Recommended Practice for Photobiological Safety for Lamps and Lamp Systems - Measurement Techniques*

ANSI / IESNA RP-27.3-2007, *Recommended Practice for Photobiological Safety for Lamps - Risk Group Classification and Labeling*

IEC 60825-1, Ed 2 *Safety of laser products - Part 1: Equipment classification and requirements*; 2007.

ISO 11146-1:2005. *Lasers and laser-related equipment – Test methods for laser beam widths, divergence angles and beam propagation ratios – Part 1: Stigmatic and simple astigmatic beams*

ISO 11146-2:2005. *Lasers and laser-related equipment – Test methods for laser beam widths, divergence angles and beam propagation ratios – Part 2: General astigmatic beams*

This appendix is not part of American National
Standard Recommended Practice Z136.4-2010,
but is included for information only.

APPENDIX

ISO/TR 11146-3:2004 / Cor 1:2005. *Lasers and laser-related equipment – Test methods for laser beam widths, divergence angles and beam propagation ratios – Part 3: Intrinsic and geometrical laser beam classification, propagation and details of test methods*

Appendix G
Measurement Pitfalls

Measurement Errors and Pitfalls.

Large measurement errors can result from a poor choice of measurement geometry and improper detector or filter selection. Therefore, it is essential to follow some basic optics principles and to consider sources of errors to obtain correct radiometric values. It is important to note that, sometimes, a possible or proposed solution may introduce other errors if proper care is not taken. Some examples of measurement errors and pitfalls follow:

1. **Problem** – the laser beam exceeds the power/energy measurement range of the detector and the radiometer reading has saturated indicating a lower power or energy than actual and creating a false sense of safety. **Solution** – simply reducing the radiometer sensitivity does not alleviate the measurement error. The entrance power or energy to the detector needs to be attenuated to operate the detector in an unsaturated mode by using an attenuating filter or limiting aperture. It may be necessary to recheck the detector calibration as damage may have occurred. Additionally, begin measurements with the new detector with significant calibrated optical density filtration in the path to protect the detector. If no signal is registered, sequentially reduce filtration until useful readings can be obtained. Alternatively, substitute a detector that includes the range being measured.

2. **Problem** – the laser beam exceeds the damage threshold of the detector and caused permanent damage to the detector. **Solution** – order a new detector. Always check the detector limits in the owner's manual, being careful to check both maximum irradiance/radiant exposure limits as well as power/energy limits. Additionally, begin measurements with the new detector with significant calibrated optical density filtration in the path to protect the detector. If no signal is registered, sequentially reduce filtration until useful readings can be obtained.

3. **Problem** – the laser beam strikes a filter and burns the reflective coating changing the filter transmission characteristics. **Solution** – discard the damaged filter and in the future stack absorbing filters with reflective filters to limit filter exposure or use reflections from a calibrated uncoated beamsplitter window to attenuate the beam before allowing it to impinge on the filters. When using multiple filters to attenuate the beam, it can be useful to stack them in increasing attenuation levels away from the beam source (i.e., Laser, ND-0.5, ND-1.0, ND-2.0) to minimize the chance of damage to the filters. Alternative solutions can include: mechanically attenuating the beam using a chopper for CW lasers; or reducing the measured beam energy or power by measuring the beam reflected from a single-surface reflector.

4. **Problem** – an attenuating filter fluoresces with the laser beam and your detector responds to this added light. **Solution** – select another filter as the first one may also be nonlinear and may actually photo-bleach at high irradiances.

5. Problem – the laser beam propagating through a stack of filters causes interference effects. **Solution** – stack filters at slight angles to each other to prevent interference.

6. Problem – the detector creates a dark current (zero offset) that has been added to the radiometer measurement. **Solution** – perform a blind-test (no applied radiation onto the detector) and measure and subtract the dark current from the reading or use the instrument zero.

7. Problem – the room lights are on and your assistant is walking around in front of the detector, or you are outdoors during daylight and experience changing cloud cover, and these changes are affecting your measurement readings. **Solution** – take measurements in the dark or at night, or from within a darkened path, or use a narrow bandpass filter passing the laser wavelength.

8. Problem – the detector was placed close to a pulsed laser that contains significant visible and/or invisible pump radiation with the laser beam. **Solution** – move the radiometer away from the laser as pump radiation falls off as $1/r^2$ (or otherwise diverges quickly) or employ a filter that blocks the pump radiation or only transmits the wavelength of the laser.

9. Problem – a pyroelectric detector is selected to make laser beam measurements in a noisy environment. **Solution** – pyroelectric detectors contain piezoelectric crystals that respond to acoustic energy and may require a blind-test to account for the error, or another type of detector should be selected. An insulating tent can be made from bubble wrap packaging material to nearly completely absorb any air pressure fluctuation or oscillation.

10. Problem – the laser system employs a bank of high-voltage capacitors that are discharged to fire the laser and the radiometer senses the changing electric and/or magnetic fields. **Solution** – perform a blind-test to ensure that the radiometer does not sense the changing fields and account for the error. It may be necessary to employ a metal screen to shield the radiometer from the electromagnetic pulse (EMP) radiation from the pulse discharges and circuit inductances.

11. Problem – a laser beam is employed to measure a filter's attenuation, but the testing setup allows forward-scattered radiation from the bench-top to bypass the filter and be sensed by the radiometer. **Solution** – install a dark tunnel between the filter and radiometer to block this scattered radiation. Seal the path between the filter(s) and the detector with opaque tape.

12. Problem – polarization of the laser beam and/or elements placed in the laser beam can cause significant measurement errors. **Solution** – check for polarization and rearrange optical components to reduce effects of polarization or make the effects known quantities and compensate for those effects.

13. Problem – the laser simultaneously emits multiple wavelengths when only one was expected. **Solution** – check for multiple wavelengths when suspected or if their existence is possible.

14. Problem – laser appears to have missing pulses because of aliasing. **Solution** – ensure the oscilloscope or radiometer sample rate is fast enough to properly detect pulses of short duration and/or high repetition rate.

15. Problem – peak power of narrow laser pulses may greatly exceed the damage level of detectors or other optical components while average power is well below it. **Solution** – estimate the peak power level and check the damage level of detectors and optical components before use. Alternatively, use calibrated uncoated beamsplitters to reflect a small portion of the beam at first and reduce peak powers to safe levels for measurements.

16. Problem – For non-uniform spatial beam profiles, the average power density may be below the damage threshold while the peak density of the profile is above the threshold. **Solution** – check beam profile and estimate peak power density, and check the damage thresholds. A couple of possible ways to compensate for this include: If laser peak/average power is below damage thresholds for an integrating sphere, use a calibrated integrating sphere and side-mounted detector for measurements. If peak/average power levels are above damage thresholds, use calibrated filtration or uncoated beamsplitter reflections to reduce power to the integrating sphere. Integrating spheres eliminate the effects of non-uniform multi-mode beam profiles.

17. Problem – background noise or radiation is below the trigger level when internal trigger is used for pulsed laser measurements, thus the effect of the background is ignored causing error in the measurement. **Solution** – use external trigger when applicable, or characterize background noise and make corrections.

18. Problem – absorptive filter may heat-up in high power applications, and consequently OD of the filter is not constant and different from that measured with low power. **Solution** – avoid the use of absorptive filters in high power laser measurements or use a filter stack. When using multiple filters to attenuate the beam, it can be useful to stack them in increasing attenuation levels away from the beam source (i.e., Laser, ND-0.5, ND-1.0, ND-2.0) to minimize this effect.

19. Problem – when using commercial power/energy meters with wavelength-calibrated sensors and attenuators, an erroneous reading may be obtained if the meter settings for the wavelength or the attenuator are incorrect. This may occur when the power meter is turned on or a different sensor head is installed, and the setting resets to a default wavelength. **Solution** – before doing the measurement, always double check that the wavelength setting corresponds to the measured laser and the attenuator setting corresponds to the actual case (ON or OFF).

20. Problem – a detector has a large correction factor (due to lack of sensitivity near the edges of its detection limits) at a particular wavelength or wavelength band, and emission at that wavelength appears substantial though a very low emission level is present. When corrected, the reading could be quite large and may, in actuality, be just an artifact. **Solution** – Ensure optimum detector sensitivity is chosen for wavelength band to minimize erroneous detector response at edges of detector sensitivity.

21. Problem – when using a power meter for high powered lasers that requires water cooling for operation, variations in the water temperature can greatly vary the output reading of the power meter, making it appear as though the laser power is oscillating when it isn't. **Solution** – Ensure that the chiller used to provide the cooling water can maintain a constant water temperature to avoid this problem.

Index